REJUVENATION!

REJUVENATION!

How the Capillary-Cell Dance Blocks
Aging while Decreasing Pain and Fatigue

Robert Buckingham, MD, FACP

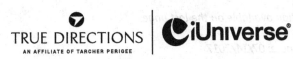

REJUVENATION!
HOW THE CAPILLARY-CELL DANCE BLOCKS AGING
WHILE DECREASING PAIN AND FATIGUE

iUniverse books may be ordered through booksellers or by contacting:

iUniverse
1663 Liberty Drive
Bloomington, IN 47403
www.iuniverse.com
1-800-Authors (1-800-288-4677)

Because of the dynamic nature of the Internet, any web addresses or links contained in this book may have changed since publication and may no longer be valid. The views expressed in this work are solely those of the author and do not necessarily reflect the views of the publisher, and the publisher hereby disclaims any responsibility for them.

Any people depicted in stock imagery provided by Thinkstock are models, and such images are being used for illustrative purposes only.
Certain stock imagery © Thinkstock.

ISBN: 978-1-5320-2276-0 (sc)
ISBN: 978-1-5320-2275-3 (hc)
ISBN: 978-1-5320-2274-6 (e)

Library of Congress Control Number: 2017906795

Print information available on the last page.

iUniverse rev. date: 07/14/2017

Contents

Contents

Illustrations

Acknowledgements

I would like to give thanks to the many people who helped support the writing of this book.

First, to my friend and professor, Dr. Radulovacki, when in medical school and as a graduate student, encouraged me to ask questions that could not be answered.

To all of my patients, each of which has helped formulate insight into inflammation in their own unique way.

To the support staff, at all the hospitals and other institutions that I have worked in, for giving me leeway to be myself to provide my own brand of care and support to patients.

To my colleagues, multitudes of them, that have been patient with my concerns and have worked with me to help solve challenging problems.

To Scott Bennett, for designing a book cover that again exceeded expectations.

To Ryan Murphy, for the effort in diligently creating the illustrations in the book.

To my adult children who continue to inspire me to reach and ponder.

To my parents and grandparents, who helped nurture a curious and reflective mind.

And to Kate, my fiance, who has given me endless support and provided light, when surrounded by dark corners.

BASEBALL AND MITOCHONDRIA?

It would seem far- fetched to connect baseball and capillary-cell mitochondria. Upon further review, there is—at least in how baseball was played by the neighborhood gang in my childhood.

In its simplest form, the boys in our neighborhood harnessed a daily effort to organize and play a modified baseball game. Figuring out how we were going to do it required creative intuition. First there was the field of weeds that required regular mowing, base paths, a pitcher's mound and backstop. Then there was the constant tweaking of game rules based on how many players could actually play that day. Playing conditions could also vary and change the rules. Playing after a rain storm with a water logged ball was very different than when conditions were dry. It did not matter though. As long as we had a cut field, one ball, one bat and at least three players, we could be out there until the sunset. It was the game that mattered. This is exactly what capillary mitochondria do. As long as they can pendulum swing their combustion, capillary cells can thrive and their game of sanitizing the interstitial space while providing for the end organ is perpetuated. Just like when our game conditions changed from day to day, capillary cell outer membrane permeability adjustments change the playing conditions of their mitochondria.

As a kid, baseball was my business. For me, it was not just about a casual glance at box scores, but an all -encompassing engrossment of baseball minutiae. Sorting all this out was a process that I would come back and forth to several times a day and well into the night. You could say that I owned baseball trivia or baseball trivia owned me. It got better as the major league baseball season matured when player home runs and runs batted in often became gaudy. When the season ended, the final numbers became incorporated into streams of consciousness, comparing and contrasting them with past and present players. The natural recourse of doing this was to create arguments with my buddies about what era and player was better. My imagination went wild.

As seasons come and go, memories fade and baseball old-timers tend to became mythical, with their .400 batting averages in a season or their 500 pitching victories in a career. Old school major league baseball parks had dimensions that exceeded 465 feet for a home run, yet Babe Ruth hit 714 of them in his career in that era! Because of changes in field dimensions, the ball, gloves and even the bats, the sport was perfect fodder for unwinnable arguments about what player or era was better. All this nuance made the sport even more interesting and addicting.

By age 11, after analyzing all of the box scores in the morning paper's sports section, armed with bat, ball and glove, I hopped on my bike and began making cold calls for the daily game. By roughly eleven AM on most days, I had rounded up anywhere between three to 18 players. Commitments were on the fly and numbers could shift based on summer vacations, chores, or family obligations.

We played our games in a wide-open field of weeds and prairie grass that we mowed into the shape of a baseball field. Our backstop was a remnant of an old swing set and makeshift chain-link fence. Bases were often gloves, and home plate could be almost anything. What mattered was the number of players. Everything else was negotiable.

We played baseball roughly from 11 AM to sunset with breaks for lunch. Game rules changed as players came and left, but play had to be suspended when our numbers dwindled to less than three. One other cause for the end of play occurred when we lost our ball in the weeds from darkness. Field conditions could change daily as a result of rain, uncut weeds, and how soggy our ball was. All of these "adjustments" required rule changes.

Most rule changes were based on the number of players who showed up to play. With fewer players, rules were amended to help the defense (those playing the field, as opposed to those batting). Adjustments included batting with only one swinging strike or hitting the ball only to a specific field of play. A swinging strike, foul ball, or hitting to the wrong field became an automatic out. Making these adjustments allowed us to continue play as our numbers dwindled. The game changed dramatically with fewer players, as hitters became more restricted in how many swings they got and where they were permitted to hit the ball.

In similar fashion capillary cells adapt to changes in prevailing conditions within their interstitial spaces. The presence of chronic inflammation in the interstitial space has the same effect on capillary-cell mitochondria as a dwindling number of players had on our baseball game. Just as fewer players created a more offensive bias in our baseball game, chronic interstitial-space inflammation causes capillary-cell mitochondria to develop a more energy combustion bias. With fewer players, our jerry rigged game increasingly handicapped the hitter in favor of the fielder. With increasing interstitial space inflammation, mitochondria increasingly handicap nitric oxide combustion in favor of energy combustion. When darkness set in, or just two players were left on the field, our game ended. With chronic inflammation, when capillary cell mitochondria continue to only combust energy, there is no rejuvenation and their numbers decrease to where the capillary cell function deteriorates and their "game" is finished.

Maybe my summers engrossed in baseball minutiae and playing baseball with my buddies with an old bat and soggy ball, on a weedy, makeshift open field, was helping me to understand how our capillary cells adapt or mal adapt to changing inflammatory conditions. And perhaps how this understanding applies to the origins of chronic illnesses, fatigue, pain, and even how we age. Except for maybe my mother, who knew.

Introduction

SOLVING THE MYSTERY OF INFLAMMATION

As a practicing physician of thirty-eight years and counting, I have come to realize that fatigue and pain are "two feathers coming from the same bird". Yet in our disease treatment models of traditional medicine they remain two of the most difficult and perplexing symptoms to diagnose and treat. The conditions they are associated with can be linked to any end organ, and often multiple end organs. And they usually involve chronic inflammation, are connected to one or more scarred up end organs and are further linked by a clustering of debilitating sometimes life-threatening illnesses. The process of diagnosing chronic fatigue and pain feels like a puzzle, where there are all sorts of pieces that appear disjointed until a few begin to line up allowing for more pieces to come together.

In is my hypothesis that most chronic fatigue and pain are a manifestation of chronic inflammation that is fueled from vascular inflammatory free radicals. Reducing these menacing free radicals will improve both fatigue and pain and cluster other benefits.

In modern clinical practice, putting the puzzle pieces together to diagnose the cause of fatigue and pain is often frustrating, time consuming, and expensive. This is because we start backwards by treating disease manifestations from end organs rather than focusing on root cause, which is inflammation. In many instances, elaborate and expensive testing or even treatment of end organ compromise may cause even more fatigue and pain and can further compromise and already dysfunctional end organ. Even when symptoms remit, they often return a short time later. Making matter worse, drugs utilized to treat pain and fatigue carry their own set of side effects, addictions and tolerances.

The big picture of inflammation usually gets lost in treating achy joints, chest pains, insomnia, anxiety, low back pain, or recurrent infections. We as consumers often just want quick solutions to our symptoms. This also usually implies skipping over discussions about our bad habits that are contributing to inflammation and our symptoms. We prefer quick in and out injections, surgery and pain medicines or stimulants and not so much the sordid details about losing weight, exercising or changing our diets. I often hear, "Just don't tell me to give up my cigarettes or lose weight, can you just give me something for the pain?" Knee jerk treatment of fatigue and pain is often the mantra of the modern 10 minute office visit to a health care provider.

Given that context, it becomes easy for practitioners to prescribe treatment for symptoms or diseases without probing the root causes of chronic inflammation. The tapestry of the underlying inflammation that produces the fatigue, aggravates pain, or contributes to shortness of breath goes unnoticed as pain killers, antibiotics, imaging studies, and expensive surgeries take precedent. Without addressing inflammation, these all become short term fixes. *Doctors don't want to spend the time, and patients may not want to hear about what they need to do to truly get better.* The medical industrial complex stands waiting at the door to take advantage of both.

Diagnosing and treating chronic fatigue and pain require a sobering awareness of inflammation and the different venues chronic inflammation utilizes to make these symptoms worse. If inflammation is ignored, regardless of diagnosis or treatment, fatigue, pain, and chronic illness return like long-lost friends.

The inflammatory stakes get higher as people get older. With aging, inflammatory risks just plain escalate without avid attention to mitigate them. With its friendship to chronic inflammation in toe, aging can accelerate with a vengeance as different vascular inflammatory free radicals stack, chronic illnesses accumulate and fatigue and pain cluster. The patient and health care provider (me included) can easily take the bait and disease treat different symptoms as if unrelated to each other. As this kind of treatment escalates there is lost ground to not only more chronic pain and fatigue, but also muscle atrophy, disrupted cognition, gait and balance, and worsening bowel and bladder control.

By age seventy, the average American is taking 6 different prescriptions, be at least fifty or more pounds overweight, has difficulty walking 6 blocks due to exertional fatigue or weight bearing joint pain, and can't consistently remember where they put their keys or parked their car. It becomes a matter of time before chronic inflammation has rendered a cancer diagnosis, disabling stroke or heart attack. It goes without saying that the epidemic of obesity has led to an avalanche of different orthopedic surgeries that include knee and hip replacements. As cancer and vascular occlusions escalate, cardiac, carotid and leg stents proliferate, imaging studies are utilized and on high demand and expensive chemotherapy is mandated for difficult to treat cancers.

Typically in the United States, surviving past 85 means graduation to walkers, wheelchairs, mechanical soft diets, adult diapers and some kind of step down care culminating in a nursing home. These bleak options carry with them two stark conclusions. One, getting old can be a nightmare and two, it does not pay to ignore the elephant in the room, chronic inflammation.

The *pain-fatigue-aging-inflammation complex*, if not addressed with about face lifestyle changes, eventually asphyxiates life without a concern for a happy ending. Besides postponing discussions about negotiating inflammatory risk, we prefer to blame others for our ailments. It's not the sugar we consume, but rather our boss, spouse or parents that made me eat the donut or box of chocolates. We formulate a system of *deserved denial*, which allows us to accept bad behavior in ourselves as a coping mechanism to mitigate the negative impact that we perceive other people, places or things have on us. Instead of facing the music head on, we prefer trading our negative perceptions about our job, boss or spouse for an excuse to snack, drink, smoke or sit. These coping mechanisms actually promote more not less inflammation and cycles more pain and fatigue, not to mention the emergence of many serious illnesses.

With combinations of denial, blaming others, and bad behavior, we dupe ourselves into thinking that the accumulation of pain, fatigue and chronic illnesses are just part of getting older. The last card played in this tragedy is fatalism, where we create a story to fit the plot of our decline. We conjure up a belief system that centers on the role of the dice, as if life's circumstances require us to yield to painkillers, cigarettes, sugar, and alcohol. Our denial and evolving phony belief system blinds us to making genuine lifestyle changes that could otherwise reverse the deep hole we are digging, aka our own graves.

Ok, you now have gotten my attention so you say. So what exactly is inflammation? A simple explanation is that it is a *cause-and-effect response* within our body to something that does not belong. The mechanism that isolates and eliminates something that does not belong is called *immune surveillance.* Both the something that does not belong and the response it creates to eliminate it causes inflammation. Chronic inflammation occurs when either the something that does not belong increases to where it cannot be eliminated or the immune response, to the something that does not belong, is inadequate or insufficient to eliminate what does not belong.

In regards to the latter, for an optimal immune surveillance response to an interstitial space of an end organ, it requires:

- a fully functioning and fluxing capillary-cell *outer membrane system*
- *on-demand raw material support* (energy, calcium ions, and nitric oxide) from capillary cell *mitochondria*
- a fully competent capillary cell nucleus with a complete set of functional *nuclear DNA* and cell infrastructure for protein repair, synthesis, and replication
- intimate communication with *end organ* and interstitial-space *mesenchymal (helper)* cells

- back-and-forth signaling by capillary cells to *inflammatory mediators(immune arsenal)* both in the blood plasma and *end-organ's interstitial space*
- communication with other adjacent capillary and downstream *large-vessel endothelial cells*
- communication with other end organs regarding hormones, enzymes and inflammatory-mediator requirements
- a full complement of *immune arsenal*

Our lifestyle choices largely determine the success or failure of how our immune system provides immune surveillance. The extent to which it fails is the same extent in which the seeds of pain, fatigue, and chronic illnesses are sown. *Rejuvenation!* dissects the mechanics of interstitial space inflammatory breach, and the mismatches that can occur involving capillary and endothelial cells, as chronic inflammation establishes an interstitial space foothold. Not to be lost in this depressing cascade is an ample discussion of how lifestyle, medicines, and supplements can set chronic inflammation on its heels by enabling a rejuvenation of capillary cell function through resetting its *dance*. The capillary-cell *dance* heretofore is defined as its outer membrane *pivoting of permeability* that is followed by a mitochondrial *swing of combustion*. It is postulated that this *back and forth pivot and swing* defines capillary cell health, which spreads to include the interstitial space, and its end organ partners.

Capillary cells are specific *endothelial cells* at the very end of the *arterial tree*; they provide a unique and specific type of support to the end-organ cells they serve. Examples of the major end organs include the heart, brain, liver, lung, and kidney. With each end organ, capillary cells have evolved a unique *outer-membrane-basement membrane morphology* to accommodate specific end-organ function. In spite of these often dramatic changes to their basement membranes, there are three constants that healthy capillary cells master control of no matter where they reside when chronic inflammation is tamed. These include refurbishment of themselves and their partners, effective immune surveillance of the interstitial space and adjustments in blood-flow and clotting dynamics. All three require optimal fluxing of permeability by capillary cell outer membranes and mitochondrial *pendulum-like shifting of combustion* to and from energy and nitric oxide. The mechanics for optimal outer membrane fluxing of permeability and mitochondrial pendulum swinging of combustion are codependent on each other. Both fail when there is chronic inflammation in the interstitial space. Throughout this book, I will refer to capillary cells separately from endothelial cells because of how capillary cells have evolved their outer-membrane morphology at such a high level to accommodate specific end-organ function.

The capacity to execute an effective immune response to prevent chronic inflammation requires capillary-cell outer membranes and their mitochondria to have intimate and optimal homeostasis with each other. The capillary cell outer membrane permeability pivot not only allows their mitochondria to decompress energy combustion but actually shifts combustion to a different production product with a different purpose. The *pendulum swing* of combustion to favor nitric oxide production creates *rejuvenation* within the capillary cell of its infrastructure, outer membranes and mitochondrial while also increasing blood flow (oxygen and nutrient) to amplify end organ function. Capillary cell mitochondrial energy combustion on the other hand facilitates immune surveillance, interstitial space sanitation and end organ rejuvenation.

Thus the push and pull of capillary-cell outer membrane permeability pivoting and mitochondrial combustion swinging from energy to nitric oxide allows the capillary cell to provide a triple function of rejuvenation and interstitial space sanitation while improving on demand end organ function. Rejuvenation also *stems* and *paces rejuvenation of* interstitial space partners that include mesenchymal and end organ cells. Said differently, mitochondrial combustion swinging allows capillary cells to effectively multitask purpose by providing the capillary cell and end organ what it needs and when it needs it. It does this, while choreographing immune arsenal to protect interstitial space hygiene. All these diverse functions are driven by the foreplay of capillary cell outer membranes and interstitial space inflammation that it responds to. As long as capillary-cell outer membranes can prevent chronic inflammation within the interstitial space by delivering the right kind, type and volume of immune arsenal, all is good within the capillary cell orbit. The avalanches of different chronic and debilitating illnesses, as well as pain, fatigue, and aging are aborted.

Anti-inflammatory lifestyles provide an unprecedented antidote to interstitial space sanitation by how they revive the capillary cell dance. With chronic inflammation, capillary cell outer membranes don't flux and mitochondrial combustion gets stuck in energy mode. Superoxide free-radicals accumulate and damage infrastructure as nitric oxide production is blocked. Without a capillary cell mitochondrial combustion swing, rejuvenation is blocked, superoxide accumulates and all things DNA get damaged. Over time, as mitochondrial volumes shrink from overheated energy combustion, capillary cells disintegrate into a dysfunctional shell.

The capillary cell meltdown is exactly what chronic inflammation desires as the door now opens for even more inflammation within the interstitial space. This occurs as immune arsenal entering the interstitial space becomes more random and mistake prone. The eventual cataclysm results in proinflammatory chain reactions, a perfect storm of converging inflammatory elements within the interstitial space. The converging inflammatory elements form an *inflammatory matrix*. With matrix formation, chronic inflammation now has enough momentum to begin setting an agenda within the interstitial space. Included in the agenda is the implementation of different mechanics that allows the inflammatory matrix more control on the space and to further isolate the end organ. If all goes to plan, the capillary cell essentially becomes a zombie, as its outer membranes are targeted for pirating by the increasingly hostile immune arsenal residing in the interstitial space. The ground work has been laid for the emergence of the *anti –organ* within the interstitial space. With the arrival of the anti-organ, chronic inflammation is now in firm control of the interstitial space and the anti-organ can now implement sets of different venues that enable chronic and disabling illnesses to emerge that further disrupt the interstitial space, isolate the end organ from its interstitial space ethos, and induce waves of clinical fatigue and pain. The progression of anti-organ venues gets very dark and include a steady torturing of the interstitial space at the expense of the end organ.

Rejuvenation! provides a *theory* on how and why we have chronic pain and fatigue, how they both relate to aging, and how the war on inflammation can be fought to win. In this theory, I introduce the capillary cell and its dance as front and center in the battle. If the dance fails, inflammatory momentum seizes up the interstitial space. If the dance continues or remerges, life is worth living for decades longer.

This theory culminates decades of carefully gathered science and a deeply intuitive perception of clinical patterns of illness based on my perch of 4 decades as an internist in the front lines of health care delivery. My hope for *Rejuvenation! is* twofold: first, to share what actually transpires within interstitial spaces before disease takes them over. And second, that I can provide a sound basis for birthing wellness into the health care equation. And now, join me as we explore the nature of inflammation and how to defend against it.

[AUTHOR'S NOTE: *Please refer to the glossary in the back of this book for a list of the clinical terminology used throughout the text.*]

Chapter 1

FATIGUE, PAIN, AND HOW THEY RELATE TO AGING

Throughout my thirty-eight years of medical practice, most patient visits involve complaints of either fatigue, pain or both. I have come to understand that they are inextricably linked by how inflammation works. Pain can cause or effect fatigue and fatigue is often linked to all types of chronic pain. Because these symptoms are so encompassing and often require different levels of urgency to diagnose and treat, the root cause(s) are easily overlooked. Far too often, the diagnosis is whitewashed in disease treatment and reduced to band aid approaches involving addictive painkillers, antianxiety medications, antidepressants, sleeping pills, muscle relaxants, or combinations of some or all of them. Often imaging and surgery are recommended but fail to control symptoms after periods of time.

While these treatments are well intentioned and offer some semblance of symptom relief, the long-term consequences of drug addiction and brain fog from untoward and addictive side effects nag a productive life. The choice is often to live with debilitating fatigue and pain, or accept the side effects, and brain fog from painkillers, antianxiety and sleeping pills. The fact is simple, all the drugs used to ameliorate pain and fatigue produce their own set of problems that can be just as bad over time as the pain and fatigue. The basis for this fact is that these medications often only relieve symptoms, can be very addictive, have their own sets of side effects and tend to lose their effectiveness over time. Remarkably they do not address the chronic inflammatory root cause(s) of pain and fatigue.

With the passage of time, as tolerance to treatments increases, even more addictive medication is required to alleviate symptoms. This creates an unrelenting spiral of potentially adverse outcomes that leave patients with even less capacity to function. Normal living gets reduced to basic subsistence and dependency upon addictive drugs. Depression, disability and suicide can be just around the corner.

Identifying the root cause is not just about which end organ is involved in the pain and fatigue complex. Although one end organ *appears to be causing symptoms*, there are usually underlying inflammatory conditions that are affecting *all end organs*. The inflammatory condition thus becomes a root cause. For example, chronic low back pain is often associated with a protruding intervertebral disc, or arthritis in joint spaces that affects nerve roots. What becomes perplexing in the treatment of low back pain is that predictability of who has the most pain based on imaging of the back is a crap shoot. Some patients have no back pain with horrific x-rays while others have severe back pain with very little evidence of arthritis. In other words, there is often no correlation between back pain and abnormalities seen on imaging. Could the difference be tied to the presence or absence of chronic inflammation?

I would suggest that any end organ pain or fatigue increases or decreases based on the presence or absence of chronic inflammation. Mitigating chronic inflammation, as root cause, has a significant impact on all types of different end organ pain or fatigue. While it is reasonable to focus resources on urgently alleviating disabling pain, the inflammatory elephant in the room should not be ignored. Identifying the root cause(s) of inflammatory pain and fatigue therefore takes on a more holistic understanding of health, as it biases discussion about anti-inflammatory lifestyles. When implemented, pain and fatigue often remit regardless of which end organ these symptoms appear to originate from. In the context of lifestyle and prevention, evaluating pain and fatigue takes on a different narrative, as reversing inflammation becomes a top priority.

In the case involving low back pain, this would mean mitigating inflammatory risks. Besides reducing dietary sugars, cigarettes, and stress, behavioral prevention programs involving low back stretching, sleep positons, as well as utilizing proper techniques in bending and lifting in aggregate substantially improve low back pain. As important as these behaviors are to addressing root cause, the fall out is that the back pain has a far greater likelihood of decreasing without relying on drugs or surgery. When lifestyle management causes a regression in pain or fatigue, patients gain greater confidence in managing their health which reinforces more wellness while making them less vulnerable to addicting narcotics or sleeping pills.

Reducing inflammation by reducing vascular inflammatory free radicals allows not only low back pain to improve but cascades occult improvements in other end organs. In the holistic, root-cause approach, the low back pain becomes the *red flag* to underlying inflammation that needs to be addressed with lifestyle adjustments. Doing so may also improve cognition, breathing and other end organ attributes.

In this chapter, we will see how the symptoms of chronic pain and fatigue tie into the cellular basis for inflammation caused by the loss of the capillary cell dance. Inflammatory influences that block this dance can be identified as those that affect the capillary cell from the *inside out*, from the *outside in*.

Outside- In Inflammation

Outside-in inflammation is caused by the macro environment we live in. These inflammatory mediators or free radicals come from the food or toxins we ingest, air we breathe, water we drink and the outside stressors that impact our emotional health and affect our sleep. Highly processed sugary-salty foods that are often packed with hidden trans-fats obliterate our intestinal microbiome, induce leaky gut, and form the foundation for serious chronic inflammation throughout our bodies. Being a couch potato, cigarette smoke, chronic alcoholism, and drug abuse all can increase risks for insomnia and stress and contribute to cascades of other chronic inflammatory conditions.

Outside-in inflammation can cluster attract and stack to accelerate inflammation when inflammatory mediator exposures link with each other. They are known as *primary inflammatory mediator risks, first-line vascular inflammatory risk factors, or vascular inflammatory free radical seeds*. They are notable in that they initiate or *seed* inflammation to endothelial or capillary-cell basement membranes and interstitial spaces. If not mitigated, they induce chronic inflammation within interstitial spaces and are linked to a persistent festering of free radical exposures. These exposures eventually induce arterial endothelial cell basement membrane thickening, increase shear (friction) within arterial lumens and separate the endothelial and capillary cell from its end organ partner.

Inside- Out Inflammation

The real damage these vascular inflammatory free radical seeds produce is from the inflammatory response they incite. That is, they *plume or expand* inflammation which is caused by the attraction of *second-line inside-out inflammatory mediators (white blood cells, cytokines)*, also known as the *immune arsenal* towards the free radicals. These second-line inflammatory mediators intervene, upon request by capillary cells, to enter the interstitial space and expand inflammation for purposes of eliminating the offending inflammatory free radical(s). If not eliminated, interstitial space inflammation festers, which can then morph into a *chronic inflammatory response*. Over time, and with the right mix of inflammatory constituents within the interstitial space, this confluence can eventually organize and take on a life of its own. It eventually coalesces to become known an inflammatory *matrix*.

The Inflammatory Matrix

One the matrix is established, chronic inflammation begins to take on its own purpose and set an agenda. Central to its agenda is to convert the immune arsenal to its own doctrine. Doing so makes the immune arsenal increasingly hostile to capillary cell intent. The matrix begins a relentless assault on interstitial space mechanics to involve both the immune arsenal and mesenchymal cells. At a critical point, the inflammatory matrix creates enough inflammatory disruption within the interstitial space that the immune arsenal begins to work against the already compromised capillary cell. Shifting loyalty of immune arsenal is key to the inflammatory matrix being able to pirate permeability control away from capillary cell outer membranes. When this occurs, the interstitial space has been locked down in favor of proinflammatory influences. Capillary cells are now sufficiently zombied, immune arsenal and mesenchymal cells confused and end organs increasingly isolated from normal interstitial space homeostasis. When this occurs, the inflammatory matrix has completed its agendas and yields to the next phase of chronic inflammation, the emergence of the anti-organ.

The Anti-Organ

With the maturation of chronic interstitial space intent, the anti-organ can appear. The interstitial space is now firmly under its domain, and means that it can now implement venues within the interstitial space to perpetuate its power at the expense of the true end organ. This usually includes generous productions of scar tissue, attempts at thrombosis, and the introduction of different types of infectious agents, cancer cells and rogue autoimmune complexes. The coup d' etat is complete when some or all of these venues establish a foothold within the interstitial space.

Therein lies the deception that chronic inflammation creates. As immune arsenal is drawn into the interstitial space, with an intended purpose to eliminate vascular inflammatory free radicals, chronic inflammation smoke screens their intent and creates confusion about their purpose. The confusion causes immune mistakes which chronic inflammation uses to further disrupt immune arsenal intent. Eventually the mistakes create so much maladjustment within the interstitial space that the immune arsenal begins to work for proinflammatory influences. This is made easier by the fact that chronic inflammation has blocked the fluxing of capillary cell outer membrane permeability which has caused their mitochondria to seriously overheat from excessive energy combustion. The overheating cascades excessive production of superoxide free radicals, which then crosslinks to disable DNA to eventually cause enough DNA damage to reduce mitochondrial volumes. As energy support for outer membrane processes involving active transport evaporates, capillary cell outer membranes pseudocapillarize their receptors, voltage gradient and pore diversity. Game on for the inflammatory matrix to now use the confused immune arsenal to pirate capillary cell outer membranes.

The persistent demands for energy by capillary cell outer membranes, for the dispersal of immune arsenal into the interstitial space to mitigate chronic inflammation, block outer membrane fluxing of permeability, which then nullifies the capillary-cell mitochondrial pendulum swinging of combustion from energy to nitric oxide. With less nitric oxide production, capillary cell don't rejuvenate and end organ cells don't get the blood flow, vis-a-vis, oxygen and nutrient they want. The triple negative means, capillary cells don't rejuvenate, the interstitial space remains chronically inflamed and end organ function becomes increasingly impaired.

By the capillary cell fluxing permeability and acting as a *stem cell* and a *pacemaker* to its partners, the mesenchymal (helper cells) and end organ cells, the blocked dance also blocks important feedback loops that contribute to both the refurbishment and function of their interstitial space partners. It would also stand that as capillary cells fail to dance, so do their partners.

Once the anti-organ gains control, its venues work in the exact opposite direction and are diametrically opposed to those of the capillary and end organ cells. The production of amyloid and fibrous scar tissue from deluded mesenchymal cells makes it very difficult for the end organ to rally or find impetus to reverse course. Already void of feedback loop relationships with the zombied capillary cells, the laying down of fibrous scar tissue and amyloid creates yet another barrier between it and the capillary cell. As capillary cells pseudocapillarize and mesenchymal cells produce scar and amyloid, end organ cells have no choice but to atrophy (shrink) to conform to an increasingly hostile interstitial space. With the advent of other anti-organ venues, it only gets worse.

As the end organ declines there are increasing waves of fatigue and pain. The anti-organ, unleashes other venues that include hiding and breeding cancer cells, infectious agents and rogue autoimmune complexes. Thrombosis and hypoxic ischemic events involving the shriveled end organ increase and further torture its existence. The anti-organ's fuel are the numerous vascular inflammatory free radicals that continue to penetrate the interstitial space. Unlike the end organ, the anti-organ can thrive with or without oxygen. Therefore it is relentless in orchestrating the activation of clotting factors and platelets within the interstitial space to cause *thrombosis*. Thrombosis is like sticking a knife into the end organ as it asphyxiates relative to the amount of blood it does not receive as a result of the clot. Thrombosis can become a slow torture to an already reeling end organ. Sometimes the torture is slow. At other times, depending on the size of the occluded artery, it can be sudden and massive.

The collapse of the interstitial space and death of the end organ could come from anyone of a number of different events, that include thrombosis, explosive cancer growth or disseminated infections. The type(s) of venues the anti-organ employs is often predicated on what genetic dye is caste within a given end organ.

Anti-organ involvement from chronic inflammation in one interstitial space and end organ is likely also occurring with different twists elsewhere. Yes, chronic inflammation in one end organ may lead the inflammatory assault, but make no mistake, inflammatory cracks are occurring in all end organ interstitial spaces. This is because chronic inflammation, and how it fuels from vascular inflammatory free radicals, knows no vascular boundaries. Chronic Inflammation is occurring in all end organs from bone, liver, intestines, adrenals, kidneys, heart, brain, eyes, ears, sex organs and lungs to peripheral nerves, smooth muscle, tendons, ligaments, cartilage and skin. Even when one interstitial space of one end organ grabs the clinical headlines with an evolving cancer, autoimmune disease or infection, the truth is there are no interstitial space or end organ boundaries from chronic inflammatory influences.

In the cases of larger arteries, their end organ cells are the *smooth muscle cells* that contract or relax actin-myosin filaments to increase or decrease blood flow by increasing or decreasing lumen diameters. Large arterial vessel involvement in the chronic inflammatory processes compounds problems for upstream capillary cells as inflamed larger vessels downstream do not provide sufficient blood flows asked for by upstream capillaries. This further stonewalls end organ interests while perpetuating those of the anti-organ.

The Proposed Pathway of Chronic Inflammation leading to the Anti-Organ

Let me summarize how chronic inflammation takes down the capillary cell dance:

- Outside-in inflammatory mediators, also known as *first-line inflammatory mediators* or *vascular inflammatory–free radicals*, increase, from a combination of lifestyle choices and genetic influences, populate within the bloodstream, migrate into the interstitial spaces of end organs, and seed to create an inflammatory response.
- As they accumulate and fester within the interstitial space, they attract inside-out inflammatory mediators, known as *second-line inflammatory mediators or immune arsenal*. These mediators are home grown which means they originate from endothelial cells, mesenchymal cells, bone marrow, lymph glands, spleen, or liver. When summoned from the blood plasma and sequenced to the interstitial space via the capillary cell they expand the inflammatory response to purpose elimination of the vascular inflammatory seed. The sequenced movement of immune arsenal (specific white blood cells, cytokines, immunoglobulins, complement and platelets), from blood plasma to the interstitial

space, is accomplished by an elaborate display of exposed capillary-cell outer-membrane receptors and supported by energy and calcium ion release from mitochondrial combustion.

- With chronic inflammation, vascular inflammatory free radicals fester and cause a persistent expansion of immune arsenal into the interstitial space.

- The festering within the interstitial space from vascular free radical seeding, that produces the persistent expansion of immune arsenal, prevents the capillary cell from downshifting outer membrane permeability. Persistent permeability energy demands then blocks the pendulum swing of mitochondrial combustion. Chronic inflammation blocks the back-and-forth fluxing of capillary cell outer membrane permeability pivot which then prevents the mitochondrial combustion pendulum swing.

- The blocked capillary cell dance, increases superoxide oxidative stress within the capillary cell as a result of excessive mitochondrial energy combustion. The accumulation of superoxide in effect overheats mitochondria, depletes antioxidants and can attach and accelerate damage to membrane surfaces and DNA.

- Capillary cell mitochondrial nitric oxide combustion decreases and with it so does rejuvenation. Capillary-cell outer-membrane receptors and burned out mitochondria are not replaced and nuclear telomeres are not lengthened. Without the capillary cell dance, not only is capillary cell homeostasis disrupted, but also that of the mesenchymal and end organ cell. The pacing of outer membrane permeability and mitochondrial combustion of capillary cell partners within the interstitial space is disrupted. This means that feedback loop driven rejuvenation to these cells is uneven or completely blocked. At this stage chronic inflammation has formed an inflammatory matrix.

- Capillary-cell outer membranes "adjust" to lost mitochondrial volumes by *pseudocapillarizing,* which means they limit their capacity to send and receive messages or to sequence an immune response. Receptors are not replaced or become silent, voltage gradients decrease or do not flux and pore diversity decreases. Pseudocapillarization makes capillary cell outer membranes ripe for inflammatory matrix pirating.

- As the outer membranes pseudocapillarize, capillary-cell permeability favors random movement of immune arsenal into the interstitial space. This creates milieus within the space for immune mistakes, thereby perpetuating even more cascades of random immune arsenal entry into the space from blood plasma. At some point a critical mass of random immune arsenal within the interstitial space becomes capable of hijacking the already disabled capillary cell outer membranes control of their permeability. When completed, the chronic inflammatory matrix turns over the keys of the interstitial space to the new sheriff-the anti-organ. This includes using the immune arsenal and mesenchymal cells towards implementing its venues.

- With anti-organ control, the interstitial space becomes ripe for fibrous/amyloid scar tissue, as well as for thrombosis, cancers, infections and autoimmune disease. Different illnesses are often predicated by end organ genetic vulnerability. As the end organ wilts from the onslaught of different interstitial space calamities, waves of fatigue and pain follow.

- All interstitial spaces of all end organs become interlocked with similar chronic inflammatory milieus.

- As multiple end-organs decline from chronic inflammation, aging accelerates.

Inflammation's Relationship to Chronic Pain, Fatigue, and Aging

Chronic fatigue and pain go hand in hand with chronic inflammation and the decline of end organ(s) function. Since chronic inflammation involves multiple end organs, although tempting, fatigue and pain should not be necessarily assigned to just one. Rather chronic inflammation involves the entire arterial tree and usually involves all end organs at some level. It could be further deduced that the level of pain and fatigue, is actually a compilation of capillary-cell failures that involve multiple end organs brought about by chronic inflammation in their interstitial spaces. The fact is that chronic inflammation produces a destructive chain reaction of clustering oxidative stress throughout the vascular system culminating in endothelial and capillary cells becoming a shell of what they once were.

Reduction in capillary-cell mitochondrial volumes caused from the blocked pivot and pendulum swing dance becomes the final straw to declining capillary-cell function. When either energy or nitric oxide production fails because of declining mitochondrial volumes, without a reduction to interstitial space inflammation, the capillary cell has no choice but to pseudocapillarize its outer membranes. When this occurs and involves declines in function of multiple end organs, not only does disease take over the interstitial space but fatigue, pain and aging become relentless pursuers.

This concept that pain and fatigue are caused from a diffuse *systemic* chronic vascular inflammatory process becomes the basis for holism. It also forms the foundation for wellness and prevention. That is chronic inflammation alters optimal homeostasis of every cell within the human body. Reversing it can restore that homeostasis thereby optimizing wellness.

Reversing pain, fatigue, and aging requires restoration of interstitial space sanitation. This mandates an *anti-inflammatory lifestyle reset*, where behaviors are put into motion to reduce *persistent seeding* of vascular inflammatory free radicals. Doing so takes the lid off capillary cell outer membrane permeability which unblocks its pivot-pendulum swing dance. Mitochondrial swinging combustion of nitric oxide drives capillary cell rejuvenation which keys reversal of chronic interstitial space inflammation. It does this by restoring capillary cell mitochondrial volumes and outer membrane receptors. This enables a return to a sequenced immune arsenal bouquet that can expertly respond to interstitial space emergencies to eliminate them. All other anti-inflammatory cascading benefits will follow.

At any given moment, the integrity of the capillary cell dance could be interrupted by the push and pull of boatloads of vascular inflammatory free radicals migrating into the interstitial spaces of end organs. Whoever or whatever controls capillary-cell outer-membrane permeability will have final say about control of interstitial space sanitation.

Root-Cause Analysis

The root cause of pain, fatigue, and aging begins with chronic inflammation and vascular inflammatory free radical seeding. The goal of the evolving chronic inflammatory matrix is to block the capillary cell dance. Without dancing the capillary cells don't rejuvenate. The immune arsenal entering the interstitial space goes from *sequenced and organized* to *random and disorganized.* All proinflammatory interstitial space momentum then follows. This is the root cause of chronic illnesses, fatigue, *pain and aging.* Cancer, infections, thrombosis, pain, fatigue, and aging become dominant clinical landscapes.

The antidote to chronic inflammation is to reverse vascular inflammatory free radical seeding in the interstitial space before chronic inflammatory venues escalate. This is accomplished by methodical reductions in the myriads of different inflammatory free radicals that penetrate and afflict the interstitial spaces and basement membranes throughout the vascular tree. Examples include tobacco toxins, AGEs (advanced glycation end products), and LDL cholesterol among others. Targeting aggressive removal of vascular inflammatory free radicals is a simple, inexpensive way of addressing root-cause of chronic inflammation.

By restoring interstitial-space hygiene, all blood vessels within the vascular tree could rejuvenate and reverse basement-membrane thickening and stabilize or reverse obstructive plaque. This reestablishes the relationship between the increasingly isolated and ignored end organ and the endothelial and capillary cell. As interstitial space sanitation improves, chronic inflammatory influences diminish as end organ functions returns.

The Victim Complex

With alarming regularity, our modern culture has enabled an unprecedented blame it on others attitude for our own bad behavior. Instead of taking personal responsibility for what we do, we blame an event, our parents, spouses, coworkers, friends, and our enemies. Consequently, over indulging in any proinflammatory activity becomes someone' else's fault. By blaming others, we become victims, allowing other people, places or things to *have control* of our bad habits. This weakens our ability to make positive changes because we don't take ownership of our behaviors.

The beginning of real change begins when we acknowledge our mistakes and take personal responsibility for our choices. In other words, to make comprehensive and long lasting change, we cannot be victims. Ownership of our behavior is the beginning of making corrections to what we do and how we do it.

Success improves when we adopt a strategy that involves those of like mind. A support system for a changed behavior is essential, and this should include spouses, family members, coworkers and friends. It means eliminating venues that nurture bad behaviors. Participating in support groups, such as Overeaters Anonymous, Alcoholics Anonymous, or Narcotics Anonymous can also be helpful. Counselors and psychologists can also lend their expertise and weigh in on methods to change behavior.

The most important step is the first one, which is to sober up and face the problem head on. See it for what it is and how it is adversely affecting your health, job, relationships, sleep and stress levels. Once the depth of destruction that the bad habit is causing is grasped, developing alternative behaviors with new support systems that limit the behavior can be implemented. Bad behaviors are typically linked to other bad habits. Anticipating the chain reactions that these behaviors create is a good beginning of getting control over addictions. Sometimes "friends" must be left behind as they can be linked to wrong choices. Whatever or whomever is part of the poor choice process must be removed to find success.

The next step involves surrounding ourselves with those who support changed behavior. As with any behavioral adjustment, there can be slippage back to old habits, but with resolve and the right kind of support, good things *will* eventually happen—and good behaviors *will* eventually stick.

Vascular Inflammation and Addictive Behaviors

Mitigating vascular inflammatory free radicals to reduce chronic inflammation can get very personal. This is because so many proinflammatory behaviors have been insidiously incorporated as habits into our daily routines. Nicotine, which is found in cigarettes, cigars, smokeless tobacco, and pipe smokers, provides an addictive foundation that requires us to smoke more over time to get the same effect from smoking. In the meantime, each time we smoke, we inhale 16 or more different toxic pollutants into our lungs which are rapidly absorbed into our bloodstream. This toxic mix not only breeds chronic inflammation in the lung, but in every blood vessel throughout the body, to eventually disrupt function in all end organs. As we age, the toxic effects becomes even more pronounced, as the combination of persistent smoking and chronic inflammation builds momentum for scarring, infection and cancer in the lung and other end organs. We often couple smoking with other pleasurable but addictive behaviors such as eating a sugary donut, candy or a burger with fries. Connecting bad habits increases chronic inflammatory momentum.

Another gateway to chronic inflammation is sugar and salt addiction. Eating just one Oreo cookie, one potato chip, or even one scoop of ice cream can lead to a feeding frenzy or several dozens of cookies, a bag of chips or a gallon of ice cream. That one cookie can also create subliminal urges for other foods or drinks with sugar. Eating just one cookie or a chip can trigger a sugar or salt chain reaction. For the next several minutes to hours we will subliminally crave more sugar or salt.

The addiction to sugar is particularly insidious. At a party or social event, one glass of wine, beer or cocktail often leads to another. As a result of a pre- dinner drink or two, we often eat more and crave more simple carbohydrates such as bread, potato or a dessert. In other words, the innocent cocktail causes us to over eat more sugar.

The next night, the relaxing and addictive pleasure derived from the previous night's alcohol can be transferred into a routine, as we cozy up to a nightly fix rationalizing the temporary pleasure derived from the nightly drink-two or three as something we deserve. What starts out as an innocent activity, becomes a permanent and escalating addiction. A similar case can be made for different street drugs, like methamphetamines or cocaine, or even prescription narcotics.

Addictions are often subliminally linked to each other based on how they cause pleasure. Hors d'oeuvres are often salty or have a variety of simple sugars in them. These sugars and salts not only increase interest in eating more than we should, but also trigger desire for other simple sugars that may or may not be sweet. This is important since we connect sugar to a sweet taste. However the majority of simple sugars are not sweet, but potentially just as addicting. Since sugar does not suppress satiety like fats do, there is always room for an after dinner dessert, sherry, piece of bread or cheese. Calories add up and weight is gained as sugar cravings increase.

Certain behaviors, such as watching TV or internet surfing, cause us to reach for snack foods like chips. Chips are salty and are full of white flour (a simple sugar), starch or both. The sugar and salt increase our desire for more as consuming one chip becomes a bag. The same is true for a late night snack. Insomnia often summons us to the kitchen for a bowl of cereal or ice cream, which can turn into consuming nightly bowls of cereal or a half gallon of ice cream.

All these behaviors cascade addictions and promote chronic inflammation. While initially appearing as harmless, over time when recurrent, produce cascades of stealth metabolic harm. As these behaviors stack with each other over time, the harm escalates at an accelerated pace.

The truly sad part of addictive behavior is how dependent we become on them. Addictions have been the cause of divorces, lost friends, children, or a job. Ending up on the street is not uncommon.

When heavily addicted and because of brain fog, chronic fatigue and pain often go unnoticed. This is ditto for the inability to recognize poor personal hygiene. Instead, all that matters is the next puff of a cigarette, snort of cocaine, 6 –pack of beer, or box of cookies. Besides, poor personal hygiene, fatigue and pain, addictions spawn early dementia and multiple other end organ declines. With rapid declines in cognition and physical endurance, permanent disability usually occurs by age 45 or even sooner. This pathetic disconnect from reality serves as a reminder as to how destructive these addictive forces are when allowed to fester.

Breaking the string of addictions requires resolve and a support system that has a better chance of success when started early, rather than before serious symptoms have set in. Support groups like AA (alcoholic anonymous), while not for everyone, have helped reverse even the most severe cases of addiction and are good places to start when there is nowhere else to go or blame. With any addiction the key behavior becomes abstinence. Getting there often requires help from many different resources.

The Ricochet of Inside-Out and Outside-In Inflammatory Mediators

As we have already learned, the chronic seeding and subsequent pluming of inflammatory mediators, blocks the capillary cell pivot and pendulum swing dance. By blocking the dance, the aggregates of increasingly random immune arsenal within the interstitial space, deflect the capillary cells' rhythm, and disable their homeostasis. This confusion centering on capillary cell rhythm, *ricochets* cascades of divergent and at times conflicting messages from their outer membranes. The ricocheted messages *block clarity and cloud intent* leading to less effective sequencing of immune arsenal entering the interstitial space. This leads to more immune mistakes within the interstitial space. The accumulation of these immune mistakes clusters even more mistakes. In this manner, a ricocheted capillary cell outer membrane signaling, caused by chronic inflammation within the interstitial space, randomizes increases in false messages leading to more immune arsenal miscues. Ricocheted messages, back and forth from the interstitial space immune arsenal and capillary cell outer membranes, are deceptive to capillary cell outer membranes and miscues additional immune arsenal being mobilized into the space. This becomes an easy way for the evolving chronic inflammatory matrix to create plumes of inflammatory disruption within the interstitial space. It eventually enables chronic inflammation to persuade interstitial space immune arsenal and mesenchymal cells to come work for it. The duped immune arsenal and mesenchymal cells become a gateway enabling the emerging anti-organ to set venues leading to viral and bacterial infections, cancer growth, thrombosis and production of scar tissue and amyloid.

The Inflammatory Endgame of Large-Vessel Obstructive Plaque

A serious outcome of proinflammatory lifestyle choices is the development of large arterial vessel obstructive plaque. Downstream from capillaries and end organs, endothelial cell basement membranes and interstitial spaces of larger arteries are adversely affected by the same vascular inflammatory free radicals that impact capillary cells. In these larger arterial vessels, the chronic inflammation on endothelial cell basement membranes can progress to thicken them and can eventually form an obstructive plaque. The plaque evolves from the chronic seeding and pluming of inflammatory free radicals and remnants of immune arsenal. Plaque growth can accelerate based on the aggregate of vascular free radicals seeds and the immune arsenal they attract towards them.

Eventually, plaque bulk applies enough pressure on the basement membrane to compress the adjacent endothelial cells. The compression compromises the vessel lumen diameter, restricting blood flowing through it. As the lumen critically narrows, the velocity of blood flowing through it decreases thereby increasing the risk for a thrombosis. If thrombosed, the large vessel occlusion produces a devastating cutoff of blood flow to upstream capillaries and end organs. Alternatively the plaque can reach a critical mass and rupture almost as if a cluster bomb. The rupture spews toxic inflammatory fragments, which can penetrate through endothelial cells and into the blood stream, to potentially thrombose and occlude smaller upstream blood vessels. Regardless of what outcome growing plaque contributes to, it can have a sudden and devastating effect to an upstream end organ.

When plaque reduces blood flow, unless there is effective collateral circulation from other large blood vessels supplying the same end organ tissue, upstream capillary cells will flail to make up the difference. Unless the large-vessel obstruction can be reversed, the end organ loses. In end organs sensitive to oxygen deficit, such as brain or heart, heart attacks, heart failure, strokes, and dementia become inevitable outcomes.

The development of downstream large vessel obstructive plaque, and the effects it has on reducing blood flow, becomes an *additional vascular inflammatory risk* to upstream capillaries. It does this by not providing enough of a blood flow response to on demand oxygen requirements from end organs. This creates predilection for nagging hypoxic inflammatory influences on upstream capillary cell outer membranes above and beyond what other chronic inflammatory influences are already causing. Large vessel obstructive plaque plays into the hands of upstream chronic inflammation and the emerging anti-organ as one more tool utilized to create malcontent within the interstitial space of the affected end organ.

The Conundrum of Inflammation and Aging

Advanced age is in itself a major risk factor to capillary-cell decline and end-organ failure. As we get older, we move, and sleep less, generally become more anxious about the world around us, and develop bad eating habits. We also lose muscle mass, get stiffer and spend more time in the bathroom either trying to defecate or urinate. All these behaviors provide fodder for increasing chronic inflammatory momentum throughout the vascular tree.

Besides all these behavioral chronic inflammatory cracks, age increases genetic mistakes in all cells. In addition, because of increasing chronic inflammation within interstitial spaces as we age, capillary cells are forced to spend more time fighting off chronic inflammatory influences and less time replacing and repairing its own constituents. In other words, age biases further blocking of the capillary cell dance.

The combination of chronic inflammation within interstitial spaces, a blocked capillary cell dance and biases towards defective DNA from free radical cross linkage, and aging produces a perfect storm for potential capillary cell futility. Because of these three inherent risks, when vascular inflammatory free radicals are not aggressively mitigated aging is often linked with aggressive anti organ venues that include relentless interstitial space scarring, thrombosis, numerous cancers and infections. Aging becomes one more risk to a blocked mitochondrial combustion swing to nitric oxide, which means rejuvenation efforts are further aborted.

Another effect linked to aging and chronic inflammation is the across-the-board reductions in endothelial and capillary cell-antioxidants, vitamins, and cofactors. All of these vital constituents are required for optimal cellular homeostasis but with aging, or the effects of chronic inflammation or both, they all diminish. In the case of antioxidants, their levels decrease from combinations of *underproduction, malabsorption, or overutilization.* The danger of diminished antioxidants cannot be overestimated. This means that more toxic free radicals like superoxide can accumulate and attach to membranes and DNA, thereby accelerating more damage. In addition, they cause more free-radical chain reactions which further accelerate aging and potentiate chronic inflammatory venues within interstitial spaces.

When the age related inflammatory equation matures, a perfect storm emerges that enables the anti-organ to rapidly escalate venues to collapse the end organ. This can and often leads to death but is also preceded by waves of fatigue and pain.

Because of age related declining DNA function and reduced antioxidants, managing chronic inflammation and vascular inflammatory free radicals in the elderly has much less wiggle room. This means that lifestyle adjustments should be more rather than less exacting, and will need to be coupled with medicinals and supplements to treat deficiency states and emerging chronic inflammatory medical issues. The goal should be to mitigate vascular inflammatory free radicals while also augmenting antioxidants in attempts to work around age related DNA damage.

Until stem cell injections become more commonplace, to perhaps reverse some of the DNA damage to endothelial and capillary cells, we must instead turn our focus on prevention and wellness.

Aging and the Push and Pull of Inflammatory Free Radicals

With age and chronic interstitial space inflammation capillary-cell outer-membrane receptors and mitochondrial volumes decrease to eventually lead to significant endothelial and capillary cell functional decline. This can remotely be compared to driving an old car. In its youth, the car would reliably start, easily accelerate upon the push of the gas pedal, stop on a dime, and get good gas mileage. With age, none of these aforementioned attributes of a newer car are as predictably reliable. At some point mileage adds up and parts age in a much older car. Even when taken good care of, it will eventually either just stop working or becomes too dangerous to drive.

The same holds true for capillary and endothelial cells. The chronic push and pull of inflammatory mediators on capillary-cell outer membranes, and the dynamic it creates to block outer membrane flux has the same effect on the capillary cell as accumulated oxidized carbon has on in an old car engine. When the car engine can no longer function, the car does not run. When the capillary cell does not perform the pivot- swing dance, it also loses its capacity to function. The reliability of a car to carry passengers to a destination is lost just as the reliability for a capillary cell to serve the end organ and protect the interstitial space is compromised.

By definition, *aging* occurs from a combination of chronic inflammation within interstitial spaces, blocked rejuvenation of the endothelial and capillary cell and its partners, and the increased genetic defects that arise within DNA from free radical cross linkage. The pace, volume and diversity of vascular inflammatory free radicals within the interstitial space that seed capillary and endothelial cell basement membranes, fuel an immune arsenal response, and block, outer membrane permeability fluxing, determines how fast capillary cell aging will occur.

Just like rust accumulating on an old broken down car, the capillary cell collapse and the emergence of the anti-organ makes the interstitial space ripe for its rust equivalent, which is scar tissue and amyloid. When a car gets old it breaks down and gets finicky. Age has a tendency to do the same thing in humans. Chronic illnesses, fatigue and pain can make getting old very difficult.

Inflammatory free radical seeding of interstitial spaces does not occur in a vacuum, will eventually cause chronic inflammation, but can be entirely preventable based upon how we choose to live. Advanced age is just a number that must be mitigated with a clean lifestyle blended with age and disease treatment appropriate medicinals and supplements.

The Pivot-and-Pendulum Effect

When chronic inflammation has been successfully mitigated by a reduction in vascular inflammatory free radicals within interstitial spaces, capillary cells are permitted to downward flux or pivot outer membranes which causes their mitochondria to *pendulum swing* combustion to nitric oxide. Ideally this fluxing pivot and swing dance between capillary cell outer membrane permeability and mitochondrial combustion is rhythmic. The going back and forth to increase or decrease permeability and swing energy or nitric oxide combustion creates healthy feedback loops that are parlayed into invoking optimal capillary and endothelial cell *quality assurance and homeostasis.* This spreads to involve interstitial-space hygiene and end-organ vitality.

The intact and fully fluxing capillary cell dance rejuvenates outer membranes receptors, voltage gradients, and pore diversity while causing replication of mitochondria to increase their volumes. Increasing capillary cell mitochondrial volumes and the energy it provides the outer membrane to facilitate active transport of immune arsenal, becomes the insurance policy that is required to minimize future risk to end-organ interstitial space chronic inflammation. The capillary cell pivot and swing dance and subsequent surge in mitochondrial volumes it causes, becomes the method of choice to prevent chronic illnesses and block chronic pain and fatigue. Capillary-cell outer-membrane permeability fluxing and mitochondrial combustion pendulum swinging are codependent, with their rhythm dependent on the third wheel; the pace and volume of vascular inflammatory-free radical seeding.

For example, in exercised skeletal muscle demands for oxygen and nutrient increase as the rate and force of actin-myosin filament sliding increases. The sliding fury requires more energy from muscle cell mitochondria. As muscle cell mitochondria call out for more oxygen and nutrient from the interstitial space the message feeds back to capillary-cell mitochondria as a powerful pendulum swing of combustion to nitric oxide. The exercised skeletal muscle not only causes nitric oxide driven rejuvenation of the capillary cell but also increases blood flow, oxygen and nutrient delivery to the interstitial space where skeletal muscle can utilize more of it. This *crisscrossing* of mitochondrial combustion and outer membrane permeability between capillary and end-organ cells is one more way capillary and end-organ cells counterbalance each other's homeostasis to each other's benefit. The capacity for this to occur is based on interstitial space sanitation and the ability of capillary cells to minimize vascular inflammatory free radicals within the space.

The brain, heart and skeletal muscle are three end organs where this crisscrossing outer membrane and mitochondrial pivot-and-pendulum effect is most obvious. In each of these, increased maximum end organ performance is directly related to how well capillary cell can deliver on-demand oxygen and nutrient. This inextricably links the crisscrossing of capillary-cell pivoting and pendulum swinging to how well the end organ's corresponding outer membranes and mitochondria respond to the crisscrossing.

"All for One and One for All"

How does chronic inflammation cascade its effects? It does so in two ways, and as such, illustrates the "all for one and one for all" integration of endothelial and capillary-cells, who rise and fall based on their aggregate homeostasis. First, outside-in vascular inflammatory free radical seeds can penetrate any end organ interstitial space. This is because many vascular free radicals can penetrate endothelial and capillary cell membrane surfaces without too much difficulty. They can also travel in stealth by latching onto to proteins that will carry them across membranes by other methods. Given their tenacity, vascular inflammatory free radicals will their way into interstitial spaces of end organs. They will figure out ways to bypass adjusted capillary cell barriers.

Once vascular inflammatory free radicals seed an interstitial space, they produce a similar pattern of pulling immune arsenal towards them. A persistently large volume of free radical seeding will likely cause chronic inflammation. When this occurs, the interstitial space has officially been red tagged!

The second way capillary cells expose the "all for one and one for all" tour de force is through their respective end organs. In this case, capillary cell homeostasis, and how well it manages the interstitial space, causes end organ function to either thrive or dive. When end organs dive the effects ripple throughout the arterial tree. The ripple includes affecting all endothelial and capillary cells and their interstitial spaces and end organs. So not only are capillary cells assaulting the same sets of vascular inflammatory free radicals in their interstitials spaces as they are elsewhere, but they are also battling levels of dysfunction from theirs and other end organs.

In this context, the decisions we make to live our lives should be reclassified as either pro- or anti-inflammatory to capillary cells. Proinflammatory behaviors accelerate declines in capillary cell and end organ function to facilitate disease treatment, whereas anti-inflammatory behaviors have the opposite effect and promote wellness.

Chapter 2

PROINFLAMMATORY RED FLAGS

Particulates, Gases, and Breathlessness

Capillary cells have adapted to specific end-organ function by modifying their basement membrane morphology. In spite of these at times dramatic changes, they still provide the same level of immune surveillance to each end organs interstitial space. Controlling interstitial space sanitation becomes the secret to enable capillary cell outer membranes to flux permeability. This becomes the mantra to the capillary cell dance and subsequent rejuvenation.

Chronic increases in inflammatory-free radical seeding of interstitial spaces will be referred to as *proinflammatory red flags*. In the lung alveolus, this manifests as a persistent inhaling of toxic gases or particulates from polluted air. Figure 19 in the appendix summarizes the normal appearance of gas exchange in a lung alveolus. With clean air and no interstitial space encumbrances, oxygen and carbon dioxide easily *diffuse* through unimpeded alveolar and capillary-cell membranes. Gases eventually meet up with circulating red blood cells, diffuse through their membranes and then attach to hemoglobin. Attached oxygen is then transported by red blood cells elsewhere to awaiting endothelial, capillary and end organ cells, where it will be utilized by their mitochondria to make energy or nitric oxide. Alveolar gas exchange with adjoining capillary cells will not be as effective when there is chronic inflammation within their interstitial spaces. Nor will delivery of oxygen be as effective elsewhere.

Chronic inhalation of particulates, whether from asbestos, various dusts, allergens, smoke, or other poisons, causes chronic inflammation of lung alveoli and adversely effects gas exchange. First, an inhaled particulate can attach to any membrane surface, including alveolar membranes to initiate an inflammatory response consisting of specific sequenced sets of white blood cells, cytokines, and immunoglobulins (see appendix, figure 20). In this example, let's use inhaled smoke free radicals. Smoke carbon particulates attach to the alveolar cell outer membranes to attract an inflammatory response, because they are foreign and don't belong there. In the figure, the inflammatory siege to eliminate them consists of neutrophils, *cytokines, IL-8 (interleukin 8), TNF (tumor necrosis factor, and macrophages.* To implement this inflammatory expansion requires capillary-cell outer-membranes to increase permeability enabling the increased recruitment, adherence, and transport of specific *neutrophils* or *(polymorphonuclear cells)* and cytokines (IL-6, 8) to facilitate containment and elimination.

The execution of the response requires capillary-cell mitochondria to combust surges of energy and release calcium ions to support active transport of a robust complement of these mitigating inflammatory mediators from the blood plasma through the capillary cell, and into the interstitial space. Unfortunately, with *chronic* smoke inhalation the sequencing response of specific immune arsenal breaks down. This is because of capillary cells exhaustion in attempting to sustain the energy effort required to provide active transport of specific immune arsenal. Without a flux of outer membrane permeability mitochondrial combustion does not convert to nitric oxide and therein lies the rub. With no capillary dance, and no rejuvenation of mitochondrial volumes, the capillary cell energy source breaks down. Pseudocapillarization soon follows and the door opens up for the interstitial space inflammatory matrix to exploit its agenda of control.

Alveolar chronic interstitial space inflammation from persistent tobacco smoke can be relentless and eventually chokes off capillary cells in providing an adequate immune response to its malingering effects. Once pseudocapillarization takes effect on capillary cell outer membranes, cascades of proinflammatory fallout follow, starting with a more random display of immune arsenal within the interstitial space.

The passive diffusion of toxic gases, including carbon monoxide, through the alveoli and into capillary cells can cause even more sinister disruption of normal gas exchange. These toxic gases can exert their own free-radical disruptions to anything they come into contact with. Because they diffuse through membranes freely they can hook up and disrupt any membrane surface of any organelle in any cell.

Once toxic gases such as carbon monoxide diffuse into red blood cells they cause a near irreversible binding to hemoglobin, thereby competitively blocking other gases such as oxygen from hemoglobin binding. By doing this carbon monoxide produces a relative hypoxia to all end organs. This can be detrimental to all end organs but particularly to oxygen sensitive ones, such as heart, brain or retina

When gas or particulate exposure is self- limiting, a brief one- time event that does not recur, capillary cells can adjust, utilize immune arsenal and mesenchymal cells to remove the noxious gas or particulate residuals and maintain a semblance of lung alveolar interstitial space sanitation. Homeostasis is maintained as capillary cells can resume the outer membrane pivot and combustion swing. All is good in the alveolar space and with its alveolar cell partners. Unfortunately, when it comes to smoking cigarettes and nicotine, this exposure is rarely just a one- time occurrence but rather a progressive and repeated pattern of addiction.

Instead, just like many addictions, smoking and the chronic inflammation it causes initially causes few if any initial symptoms. By working in stealth, it can set up a chronic inflammatory network within alveolar interstitial spaces that can become quite organized to even precipitate anti-organ venues before it is even recognized. Besides cough, occasional chest pain, breathlessness and exertional fatigue, the anti-organ forays different combinations of thrombosis (clots), asthma, scarring (emphysema), infections (pneumonia), and cancer. The medical industrial complex is ushered into the picture as symptoms build. These include frequent emergency room visits for cough and breathlessness, expensive and repeated imaging studies, a cadre of different invasive procedures that include biopsies and surgery, and the chronic use of several different kinds of inhalers, oxygen, nebulizers, steroids and antibiotics. Symptoms come and go but mostly progress regardless of the intervention. Life soon gets reduced to an oxygen cord, an around the clock medicine time table, chair, bed, and bathroom. Getting out and about usually means a trip to the doctor, pharmacy or cancer center.

The key is to recognize the malignant intent of smoking before too much damage has occurred. This is hard, since inhaled nicotine is very addictive, pleasurable and there are few if any annoying symptoms early on. This actually becomes the signature statement about addictions. In the early stages they don't cause symptoms and provide pleasure. When they do cause symptoms, chronic inflammation has already substantially impaired the capillary cell dance. The best approach to addictions is abstinence.

With tobacco smoke, proinflammatory effects are not just compartmentalized to the lung. The sixteen different contaminants easily find their way into the blood to harass membranes and interstitial spaces everywhere. Rather, the inflammatory risk meets and greets endothelial and capillary cell in the body to eventually disrupt every end organ.

The Sugar Inflammatory Assault

Sugar and smoke produce an incredibly potent one –two punch of addictive and multiple proinflammatory free radical seeds affecting all endothelia and end organs. As such they are both considered gateways to multiple addictions and accelerators of chronic interstitial space inflammation. Simple sugars come in multiple forms, are highly addictive, and do not have to be sweet tasting. All of these so called simple carbohydrates have no effect on *satiety*, meaning they don't block a desire to eat more than we should. Making matters worse, they increase cravings for more sugars. This craving can be subliminal in that we aren't aware that the food we choose to eat is being chosen because of its sugar content. Couple subliminal craving with blocked satiety and there is a recipe for obesity.

Sugars are abundant in not only things tasting sweet, but in most processed foods that involve wheat, rice, yogurt and dairy. This group would include most pre-packaged snack foods that double down on addiction by adding salt for more taste.

When it comes to package labeling, sugar grams can be deceptive as only certain simple carbohydrates are required by law to be called sugars. This means that labels can hide the actual quantity of sugars by not including them in the sugar category. So most prepackaged and processed food has much more simple carbohydrate in the product then what is actually labeled. This deception at first blush appears innocent, but in reality it produces a disturbing uptick in sugar grams of most processed foods.

Simple sugars or simple carbohydrates include table sugar, known as sucrose, as well as lactose (found in dairy), fructose (found in the very sweet fructose corn syrup), galactose, maltose, sorbitol and alcohol sugars. All of them are subliminally addictive to each other, block satiety, and can contribute to multiple proinflammatory free radicals.

Since ingesting sugars disturbs the intestinal microbiome and rushes simple carbohydrate to the liver a variety of proinflammatory cascades soon follow. When sugarholic behaviors persist, chronic interstitial space inflammation increases. In the liver, this causes transition of liver cells to become more like fat cells in what is known as fatty liver. The fatty liver changes cascade multiple proinflammatory free radicals that include elevated blood sugars, AGEs (advanced glycation end products), LDL cholesterol, triglycerides as well as elevations in highly sensitive C-reactive protein (HSCRP). All of these interfere with the endothelial and capillary cell pivot and swing dance.

When I say, that simple sugars subliminally increase addiction to each other, it means that lactose an unsweetened sugar found in dairy when consumed could increase cravings fructose, a sweet sugar found in corn syrup. When yogurt contains lactose, sucrose and fructose, it becomes a very addictive concoction. When chosen for breakfast, it could substantially increase sugar cravings that subliminally influence food choice for the rest of the day. This could include a cookie for lunch, fruit for a mid- afternoon snack and a glass or two of wine at night with some cheese. In this way, dipping into a can of fruit cocktail, which is abundant in fructose corn syrup, will manufacture cravings for chips (white flour), bread, cereal, desserts, fruit or alcohol.

When I say sugar becomes a gateway to other addictions, it means that the pleasure of eating a donut or having a dessert after dinner is often coupled with smoking a cigarette or having an after dinner drink. The donut or dessert could increase the risk for tobacco or alcohol addiction.

When sugars are chronically ingested in large amounts, weight is gained, diabetes escalates and hypertension and elevated blood LDL cholesterol and triglycerides become epidemic reminders of multiple vascular inflammatory free radical influences. As livers turn fatty and adipose accumulates in our protuberant abdomens, our metabolism becomes an eyesore. The coupling of so many vascular inflammatory risks escalates interstitial space inflammation at an unprecedented pace thereby cutting off the capillary cell dance and enabling the emergence of chronic inflammatory agendas in all end organs.

The combination of excessive ingestion of sugars, coupled with weight gain and lack of exercise breeds adult diabetes. Adult-onset diabetes (type 2 -diabetes) is defined as a fasting blood sugar of greater than 125 mg/dL or a hemoglobin A1C of greater than 6.4. *Prediabetes* (also called *insulin resistance*), often predates a transitioning to diabetes and is also vascular inflammatory, is defined as a fasting blood sugar of 101–125 mg/dL or a hemoglobin A1C of 5.7–6.4. Adult-onset diabetes is in contrast to *juvenile diabetes mellitus (type 1- diabetes)*, where the pancreas does not produce enough insulin to support glucose metabolism. Discussions from here on out will only involve the much more common adult-onset diabetes.

Adult-onset diabetes typically transitions from prediabetes, as elevated blood sugars parallel increases in weight, inactivity and loss of muscle mass. These changes often coincide with a similar liver *hepatocyte* transitioning to become more like a *fat cell (fatty metamorphosis)*. When liver cells transition to fat cells they sicken, as they lose much of their manufacturing and distribution diversity for synthesis of proteins, clotting factors and other vital constituents that other end organs need. Fatty liver metamorphosis represents a chronic inflammatory transition that can eventually leads to cirrhosis (scarring) of the liver.

One of the many ways in which diabetes creates inflammatory chaos within cells including capillary cells is how they affect *energy substrate, mitochondrial combustion, glycolysis and gluconeogenesis*. Adult diabetes causes mitochondria to utilize *fatty acids over pyruvate* to make acetyl coenzyme A. Utilizing fatty acids to make acetyl CoA creates an extra metabolic step(s) that potentially increases superoxide free radical exhaust. The subtle increase in superoxide exhaust over time increases the risk for damaging membrane surfaces and DNA.

In addition, as fatty acids are utilized to produce acetyl co A, pyruvate subsequently is underutilized and builds up in the cell, feeds back to the gluconeogenesis apparatus in the cytoplasm, and increases the production of glucose. This glucose eventually enters the blood stream and elevates blood sugars, and creates opportunity for free radical -advanced glycation end products, all while exacerbating liver production of LDL cholesterol and fat production of triglycerides. The perpetual mitochondrial combustion of fatty acids at the expense of pyruvate to make acetyl co A in all human cells self- perpetuates a vicious proinflammatory cycle.

Adult-onset diabetes increases in the elderly as skeletal muscle mass and exercise levels decrease, sleep becomes deprived and diets become more fast food. In fact hemoglobin A1C levels tend to increase over time and with age in most adults. The risk escalates further as weight is gained and obesity (body mass index [BMI] greater than 30) is diagnosed. Other risks to adult diabetes include a strong genetic family cohort for diabetes, persistent stress, and certain medications.

When adult diabetes also includes obesity, elevated LDL cholesterol, and hypertension, it becomes known as *metabolic syndrome*. This term identifies a clinical entity that is linked to a rapid escalation of chronic interstitial space inflammation. The metabolic syndrome means that a perfect storm of inflammatory mediator free radicals involving multiple different inflammatory mechanisms are working together to block the endothelial and capillary cell dance.

The loss of skeletal muscle mass from aging and inactivity has a devastating effect on how the body utilizes energy substrate, which in turn regulates blood sugars. As muscles atrophy, they lose both filament thickness and mitochondrial volumes. This combination reduces the capacity of muscle to use energy substrate (pyruvate or fatty acids) when skeletal muscle is exercised. With less utilization of energy substrate, insulin resistance increases. Figure 27 in the appendix demonstrates the normal anatomy of a muscle fiber. The loss of actin and myosin filament thickness and mitochondrial volumes in skeletal-muscle cells reduces their tone and capacity to utilize energy substrate. The buildup of blood sugars and fatty-acids in the blood from less skeletal muscle utilization becomes a red flag for diabetes.

The effects of elevated blood sugars, especially from ingestion of sugars, produces multiple vascular inflammatory free radical seeds that effect endothelial and capillary cell basement membranes, the homeostasis and exhaust of mitochondrial combustion of acetyl CoA, and the subsequent overutilization of gluconeogenesis. The clustering of these proinflammatory effects push the interstitial space anti-organ agenda and subsequent venues that ripple through the interstitial space immune arsenal, mesenchymal and end organ cells throughout the body. All together they unleash a pluripotent stemming of inflammation that accelerates interstitial space chaos and anti-organ emergence.

It takes a lot of wherewithal to defeat the many splendored sugar demon. It begins with recognizing that all sugar is not sweet and that there are hidden sugars in many foods that go unaccounted for on their labels. Then it requires an understanding of transactional cravings and misguided subliminal urges. This makes the sugarholic an occult proinflammatory menace because in most instances we are not aware of the degree to the inflammatory assault. Being not aware, and because of the pleasure that ingested sugar causes, makes it is easy to relapse to its addiction and subliminal cravings. Having a constant lookout for potential sugars will help. Knowing how highly processed and fast foods feed the cravings by adding salt is important. The most important thing to remember is that sugar does not need to be sweet to be deadly.

Gum Disease

Chronic periodontal gum disease (chronically infected and receding gums) is attributable to an altered mouth microbiome which is perpetuated from a combination of secreted salivary enzymes and abundant vascular inflammatory-free radicals. Receding gums contribute to tooth decay, periodontal abscess, tooth loss, and chronic mouth pain. It is caused from chronic inflammation within the interstitial spaces of the gums, which allows the anti-organ to create a venue enabling the penetration of bacteria. Once bacteria penetrate the gum line in earnest, the gum interstitial space has been firmly coopted by anti-organ influence. The bacteria can populate the interstitial space to cause a gum abscess or migrate through the disabled capillary cell and into the blood stream and set up shop elsewhere, such as in cerebral or coronary artery or heart valve. Bacterial gum disease becomes dangerous to the brain and heart.

Besides metastasizing serious interstitial space inflammation elsewhere through bacteria spread, periodontal gum disease causes malodorous breath, disrupts chewing, limits what kind of food we can eat, and contributes to dysfunctional swallowing and food aspiration into the lungs. It can be a source of chronic mouth pain and potentially increase risk for gum cancer. Chronic glum disease can also spread locally to cause maxillary sinusitis and even brain abscess. Gum disease can be perpetrator of chronic fatigue.

The gums are composed of *epithelial cells* that provide barrier support to teeth roots from mouth salivary enzymes, food, and bacterial microbiome. The mouth, just like the intestines, has an optimal *bacterial microbiome*, which supports mouth homeostasis and mastication. The microbiome is improved by the ingestion of plant fibers, supports salivary enzymes in the initial processes of mastication and nurtures gum interstitial space health by limiting what I call *leaky gum*. Leaky gum affects the quality of salivary gland enzyme excretion. Sugary diets alter the mouth microbiome and increase risk for leaky gums by disrupting salivary gland secretions. Eventually tis will open the door to chronic interstitial space gum inflammation. Chronic glum inflammation blocks the capillary cell dance thereby enabling the eventual emergence of the anti-organ and the venue of bacterial penetration into the interstitial space. Chronic gum interstitial space inflammation, has its origin in a leaky gum, is exacerbated from an altered mouth microbiome and triggered by a sugary diet. As such it becomes a red flag to chronic periodontitis and all the inflammatory fall-out that follows.

Sugary diets are not the only way that the microbiome can change in the mouth. Adult diabetes, tobacco smoke, chewing tobacco or drug-alcohol abuse can have similar effects as sugar. It becomes only a matter of time when one or any of these vascular inflammatory free radicals risks creates enough leaky gum for chronic inflammation to emerge the anti-organ, pirate capillary cell outer membranes and cause the emergence of invasive bacteria within the interstitial spaces of the gum. With the capillary cell disabled, it becomes not if but when they spread elsewhere.

The expense of managing chronic periodontal gum disease can be exorbitant with the simplest of solutions to just pull all the teeth. Anything else and expenses escalate substantially as root canals and expensive dental implants can cost in the tens of thousands.

On the other hand early reversal of vascular inflammatory free radical risks postpones or prevents much of this periodontal quagmire. By restoring an optimal mouth microbiome and taking other measures to prevent gum atrophy capillary cells in the gum line are enabled to dance, flux permeability and swing combustion. This enables a return of interstitial space sanitation and pushes the anti-organ and it avenues into reverse isolation. Doing so reverses the deadly anti-organ push of what could be construed as a bacterial dissemination of a *systemic vascular disease to the brain and heart vasculature.* Lifestyle choices, with particular reference to more plant fiber and less sugar, but also to include avoidance of tobacco, drugs and alcohol, can prevent the leaky gum. Prevention techniques, such as regular brushing, flossing and regular professional teeth cleaning also play an important role. By avoiding gum disease, your heart, brain, and kidneys will thank you.

"Leaky Gut" Syndrome

Chronic inflammation within the interstitial spaces of the intestinal tract leads to *"leaky gut"* which is defined as missteps in nutrient passage into the portal venous circulation. Leaky gut induces toxic malabsorption, as it causes preferred nutrient to leak back into the intestinal lumen, while at the same time allowing more toxic constituents, entrance into the portal circulation. Leaky gut begins with an altered intestinal bacterial microbiome and is perpetuated by a sugary diet and chronic vascular inflammatory-free radical seeding within the intestinal interstitial space. It becomes a propagator to chronic inflammation the eventual emergence of the anti-organ and a springboard of different venues that contribute to various chronic and serious illnesses within the intestinal tube. These include a full spectrum of different presentations, from erosive bleeding events to the development of various diarrheas, thrombosis, infections, cancerous polyps and autoimmune disorders. As such, leaky gut red flags chronic intestinal tract inflammation, eventually leads to multiple serious intestinal tract outcomes, and become the origin of intestinal tract related pain and fatigue. The absorbed toxic nutrient cascades inflammation to involve the functioning of multiple capillary cell beds and end organs elsewhere.

Leaky gut has its origins in fake or highly processed foods. Fake food is usually engineered, highly processed, addicting, loaded with sugar and salt, and contains few if any antioxidant. It is the antithesis to eating fresh vegetables. Processed food almost always has either the simple sugar lactose or the protein gluten linked with it. Both of these constituents can increase abdominal bloating, gas and diarrhea in those intolerant or with increasing age. Figure 21 in the appendix demonstrates the relationship of capillary to intestinal epithelial cells in an *intestinal crypt*. The crypt helps to exaggerate exposure of intestinal epithelial cells to the bacterial microbiome in the lumen, thereby providing greater surface area for their interaction and subsequent nutrient absorption. Different intestinal epithelial cells specialize in absorbing different nutrients and electrolytes. This is improved when the intestinal microbiome is upgraded by a plant based diet. By upgrade I mean that eating fresh vegetables improves the quality of bacteria populating the intestinal microbiome. Better bacteria mean less leaky gut, which translates into less toxic nutrient exposure within the interstitial space, less risk for chronic inflammation and less blocked capillary cell dancing.

The quality of nutrient handoff from the microbiome to the intestinal cell epithelium is a critical feature in preventing leaky gut. If nutrient is not packaged properly, or the handoff includes ingested toxins, excessive sugars, nitrosamines or trans- fats, leaky gut can be exaggerated and chronic inflammation in the intestinal interstitial space more likely.

Simply put, leaky gut increases Intestinal chronic inflammation and malabsorption, disables the capillary cell dance and allows anti –organ preeminence in the interstitial space. Besides increasing all its venues within the intestinal tract its effects are also felt systemically. These include combinations of chronic fatigue, achy joints and muscles, skin rashes, kidney filtering issues, liver inflammation, and varying levels of brain fog.

Can an anti-inflammatory diet rich in plant fiber change the microbiome, reverse leaky gut and improve control of interstitial space vascular inflammatory free radicals? The answer is an unqualified yes. Mounting evidence is irrefutable that diets with a *lower glycemic and higher vegetable fiber index,* such as the *Mediterranean diet,* decrease chronic intestinal interstitial space inflammation and all the fall-out that follows.

Fatty Liver

With combinations of fresh vegetable fiber an optimal microbiome, and a reduced circulating vascular inflammatory free radical burden, intestinal epithelial and capillary cells will optimize delivery of an exceptional nutrient package into the portal vein circulation. This package is delivered by the portal vein to capillaries in the *liver sinusoid* (see appendix, figure 23). Blood arriving from portal veins makes up 70 percent of total blood flow to the liver sinusoid, with the remaining 30 percent commixed with hepatic arterial blood. This creates a mixture of both nutrient and oxygen rich blood arriving to the liver sinusoid.

A liver sinusoid consists of well-organized clumps of liver cells (*hepatocytes*), an interstitial space (*space of Disse*), flat and very porous capillary cells, and mesenchymal cells within the space of Disse (*Kupffer* and *stellate* cells). As blood flows through the sinusoid (flowing from left to right in figure 23), nutrients are barely filtered through porous capillary cells to then enter the interstitial space of Disse. Nutrient is then washed up against awaiting hepatocytes, where it is rigorously engulfed into the cell through a variety of different mechanisms. Once in the hepatocyte, nutrient and oxygen are utilized as substrates for liver manufacturing and distribution of glycogen, energy substrates, different proteins, inflammatory mediators, clotting factors, and cholesterols. At the same time, liver cells secrete bile (flowing right to left in the figure), which facilitates processing of fat molecules. Bile drains into its own duct system (*bile ductule*) to eventually enter the common bile duct. Bile is stored in the gallbladder, released with ingestion of a fatty meal, and travels through the common bile duct to the small intestine where it is then utilized to catabolize fatty nutrient. Figure 24 in the appendix shows a magnified view of the liver sinusoid, with a row of hepatocytes, the interstitial space of Disse, a Kupffer cell within the space, and capillary endothelial cells.

Besides its extensive manufacturing activities, the liver hepatocytes also packages fatty acids, which are shipped to abdominal *adipose cells* (fat cells) for further processing and storage. The liver cells also participate in the detoxification of many different drugs, alcohol or other ingested or acquired poisons. They do this with an array of different enzymes that break chemical bonds while adding or subtracting carbon, phosphate, hydrogen, and nitrogen atoms.

Disruption of this intricate display of alchemy by liver cells can occur from chronic inflammatory influences that disrupt the space of Disse. The risk for chronic inflammatory confusion within the space of Disse is compounded by the porous nature of capillary cell outer membranes, which allows for a broad spectrum of potential blood plasma inflammatory exposures. These exposures would include the presence of circulating bacteria, viruses, or cancer cells. The potential for chronic inflammation within the space of Disse is therefore magnified compared to the interstitial spaces of other end organs. It also makes the *patrolling* rolls within the space of Disse, the Kupffer and stellate cells, critical partners to immune surveillance. It becomes there job to pluck unwanted cells, bacteria, viruses and particulates out of the space, and either auto digest them, or ship them back to the capillary cell before they enter the hepatocyte.

As in other end organs, with chronic interstitial space of Disse inflammation, the capillary cell pivot and swing dance is blocked. With persistence and progression of inflammation, constituents involved with inflammatory momentum within the space coalesce to produce an inflammatory matrix. An organized inflammatory agenda which further disorganizes the interstitial space is set into motion with similar patterns of influence as in other end organs interstitial spaces. As immune arsenal, Kupffer and stellate cells are duped to switch sides, the capillary cell outer membranes become subject to an increasing array of mixed and confusing messages coming from the interstitial space. Already partially disabled from combusting too much energy, capillary cells become ripe for inflammatory matrix pirating of outer membrane permeability channels. When this occurs, the space of Disse anti-organ emerges, and begins to set venues within the interstitial space. One venue to for the production of scar tissue or amyloid from duped mesenchymal cells. Other venues plan for the emergence of different infections, cancer or autoimmune disease. While this is occurring, the capillary cell mitochondrial volumes have shrunk to critically low levels and their membranes have pseudocapillarized, thereby opening the door for a complete takeover of the by now hostile interstitial space of Disse immune arsenal.

As chronic inflammation sets its own rules within the space of Disse, the sinusoidal hepatocyte feels the pain and transitions to become more like a fat cell. This produces a dramatic change in how the liver cell functions, and is known as *fatty liver metamorphosis*. As inflammation continues, liver cells will continue to transition. In addition to becoming fatty, they can eventually atrophy as stellate cells produce more fibrous scar and amyloid. This late transition stage of the hepatocyte, which is dominated by fibrous scarring and liver cell atrophy, is called *cirrhosis*.

When liver cells decline, there bad fortune cascades to involve multiple other end organs. With combinations of deficient clotting factors, inflammatory mediators, circulating albumin, coupled with the buildup of ammonia in the bloodstream, malnutrition, cancer, bleeding, blood clots, infections (sepsis), leg edema, compromised kidney filtering, and brain fog escalate. Muscle sarcopenia, fatigue and pain increase. The abdomen distends as it becomes full of fluid, known as *ascites, which becomes a breeding ground for infections, cancer, clots and bleeding.*

Figure 22 in the appendix depicts a cross section of a capillary cell from the liver sinusoid. Unlike other capillaries, capillary cells in liver sinusoids have basement membranes containing large gaps (*fenestrae*) that lack diaphragms. These membrane gaps provide adjacent liver cells, across from the space of Disse, more or less direct access to portal vein and arterial blood. Figure 16 in the appendix further depicts these features, comparing the "wide-open" capillary cell outer membrane in the liver sinusoid (on the far right) to what might be seen in the intestines (middle) and then what a capillary cell would look like in the blood-brain barrier (far left). Capillary cells in the liver sinusoid, in contrast to anywhere else, offer the liver hepatocyte cell unmatched exposure to blood plasma constituents but at a price.

Key to space of Disse sanitation is a clean blood plasma with reduced vascular inflammatory free radicals. This permits capillary cells within the liver sinusoid capable of the fluxing pivot and swing dance, which sets up the capillary cell to succeed in immune surveillance of the interstitial space of Disse. The pivot and swing dance enables capillary cells shift combustion to nitric oxide thereby certifying their rejuvenation while pacing similar activities to their space of Disse partners.

Like a self- repeating broken record, it starts by an optimal plant based diet and spreads to include exercise, sleep hygiene and stress management. Enabling the capillary cell pivot and swing prevents the liver sinusoid hepatocyte from transitioning converting to a fat cell, thereby preventing the gateway to other serious liver outcomes.

Filtering Malfeasance

Capillary cells within the kidney *nephron* form a unique filtering relationship with specialized epithelial cells called *podocytes*. They clump together to filter blood plasma in a capsule-like structure known as a *glomerulus*. In a normal kidney, there are as many as one million nephron units, each containing a glomerulus. Initial filtering in the glomerulus produces an *ultrafiltrate*, a process whereby waste products are removed from the arriving blood plasma while proteins and other blood constituents are bypassed to recirculate in the blood stream. The ultrafiltrate then passes from the glomerulus to a series of collecting tubules that further refine the ultrafiltrate by removing electrolytes and water. This creates the final product, known as *urine* (see appendix, figure 25). The urine empties into a *renal (kidney) pelvis* and then drains into a long *ureter* tube, which empties into a retaining sac known as the *bladder*. Urine leaves the body from the bladder by traveling through another tube, the *urethra*.

The capillary-cell outer membranes contribute to the initial filtering process in the glomerulus by utilizing active (requiring energy) and passive (not requiring energy, also called diffusion) transport processes to remove waste products, electrolytes, water, and minerals (see appendix, figure 26). The figure depicts capillary cells in cross section, showing their large pores and thick basement membrane. To compose an ultrafiltrate, the blood plasma must pass through four membranes (two each from the capillary and podocyte cells) in the glomerulus. What can't be seen in the figure is the narrow interstitial space between the capillary-and podocyte cell, which is where chronic inflammation can disturb glomerular filtering.

The chronic festering of vascular inflammatory free radicals, toxins, and inflammatory debris within the interstitial space of the kidney glomerulus can induce a chronic inflammatory stew that menaces the filtering process. The inflammatory stew blocks the capillary cell pivot and swing dance by invoking chronic pressure on capillary cell membranes to transport immune arsenal into the space to neutralize the persistent inflammatory free radicals. Over time this creates the same pattern of capillary cell dysfunction as has been reported previously. Eventually inflammatory momentum within the interstitial space organizes to form an inflammatory matrix, set an agenda, and a new set of rules within the space. The new rules run counter to capillary and podocyte filtering and eventually sicken the capillary cells to a point where they pseudocapillarize their membranes from the loss of mitochondria. Enter the anti-organ and its sinister array of venues. Glomerular interstitial space scarring, thrombosis, infections, autoimmune-complex disease, or cancers are all part of the proposed anti-organ agenda.

The anti-organ agenda(s) cause serious declines in the quality of the ultrafiltrate. A lot of what should be filtered isin't and that which is removed shouldn't be. In other words, the ultrafiltrate isin't really anything close, as the capillary cell driven processes of waste removal have been severely disrupted which has cascaded to also involve similar processes on the podocyte side. Much of this disruption is caused by inflammation on the capillary cell basement membranes which has been the primary driver of the blocked capillary cell dance. As the ultrafiltrate declines blood plasma poisons are not removed, electrolytes are not rebalanced, acid base balance is disrupted, and albumin proteins are lost. The filtering disruption produces cascades of proinflammatory waste buildup in the blood plasma, that when coupled with electrolyte, protein and acid- base mismanagement, adversely affect endothelial, capillary and end organ cells elsewhere.

The initial festering leading to glomerular interstitial space inflammation can be set off my different inflammatory entities but is accentuated by the presence of vascular free-radical "seeders". These can include the usual culprits, AGEs, LDL cholesterol, various toxins and drugs, stress hormones, and other poisons, among others. In aggregate, these free radicals invade the interstitial space by penetrating often in stealth through the ineffective capillary cell shield. Once in the space, rather than continue their voyage through the podocyte, they harbor within the interstitial space, attach to membrane surfaces and attract immune arsenal from the blood plasma towards them. This perpetuation of chronic inflammation within the interstitial space is the mechanism that silences the capillary cell dance to eventually kill glomerular ultrafiltration. As filtration fails and the blood becomes a poisonous bath, respirations increase, heart rhythm disturbances that could induce sudden death become common, brain fog to the point of stupor is elicited, and waves of fatigue and pain become commonplace within the clinical landscape. In later stages, fluid retention, brittle bones, sleep disturbances, elevations in blood pressure and both respiratory and heart failure increase.

This brings us back to the anti-dote to glomerular filtering malfeasance: "lifestyle, lifestyle, and lifestyle". Anti-inflammatory lifestyle choices reduce vascular inflammatory free radical seeding of the glomerular interstitial space, which cracks open the door that enables capillary-cell outer membranes to downward their permeability to immune arsenal. This permeability downdraft reacts favorably to capillary mitochondria, which then push combustion towards nitric oxide. This combustion shift reawakens the capillary cell from its zombie snooze to stir nitric oxide driven rejuvenation. With the capillary cell back in business, the control of interstitial space momentum shifts back to the capillary cell-end organ axis. The kidney glomerulus comes back to life and the ultrafiltrate actually ultrafilters. The momentum swing in interstitial space control causes both mesenchymal cells and immune arsenal to once again reverse course and ally themselves with once again to the "good forces". Improved interstitial space sanitation means that the anti -organ has been placed in reverse isolation. Weakened but not forgotten, it can and will reemerge given the right set of circumstances.

Dementia

Capillary cells of the brain and spinal cord are critical to the optimal function of nerve cells. In direct contrast to liver sinusoidal capillaries, brain and spinal cord capillary cells create a potent barrier (known as the *blood brain barrier*) between blood plasma and brain tissue. Only very select nutrient, oxygen, electrolytes, minerals and proteins get access to the brain, as its cells are bathed by a clear colorless nutrient enriched fluid known as *cerebrospinal fluid*. Blocking or at least limiting access of most blood constituents helps prevent nerve-cell damage while optimizing their function.

Composed of a cell body, nucleus, dense mitochondrion, other organelles, axons, dendrites, and outer membranes, nerve cells are highly specialized electrical and chemical conduits. By generating rapidly firing electric currents through their dendrites and axons and secreting chemical neurotransmitters they rapidly transmit messages to specific bundles of adjacent nerve and glial cells, while constantly messaging oxygen and nutrient demands to capillaries of the blood brain barrier. Capillaries respond to these messages by pivot and swing dancing, to enable their mitochondria to increase or decrease combustion of either energy or nitric oxide. Whereas energy combustion either keeps immune arsenal in or out of the brain bath to maintain its pristine sanitation, nitric oxide production both rejuvenates the capillary cell while providing an essential blood flow backdrop enabling rapid adjustments to regional brain blood flow. This provides the basis for the brains ability to adjust its different sets of complex cognitive functions. As brain cells are stimulated to work, they simply need more oxygen and energy substrate to facilitate electrical charges and release of neurotransmitters. Bringing in more on- demand blood flow, with more oxygen and nutrient, becomes the answer.

Nerve cells could not survive without the blood brain barrier. The barrier is essentially a highly specialized immune-surveillance support system. In normal conditions, it only allows blood plasma immune arsenal access into the cerebrospinal fluid when there is a need for them. This unique barrier arrangement serves as insurance that the immune arsenal cannot have easy access to nerve cell outer membrane, axon or dendrite surfaces that could trigger an autoimmune complex reaction. Figure 16 in the appendix to the far left, demonstrates capillary-cell outer membrane of the blood brain barrier. Capillary cells of the blood brain barrier are tightly compacted with tight gap junctions and no basement membrane gaps. The resultant cerebrospinal fluid-bath serves as a nutrient, electrolyte, mineral and oxygen bath while also facilitating a perfect conduit medium for the movement of electrical impulses.

The blood brain barrier is actually a *unit,* composed of capillary cells, *pericytes,* and *glial-astrocytes* (see appendix, figure 15). The corresponding figure demonstrates the transitioning of the larger arterioles, surrounded by smooth muscle, to the more fragile capillary cells, which lack smooth muscle. The capillary cells, with the help of specialized partner cells, astrocytes and pericytes, form a wall to seal the border between blood plasma and the brain's infrastructure.

Barrier support requires more energy from capillary cell mitochondria to execute active transport processes (exocytosis), to push unwanted molecules back into the circulation. Hence capillary cells of the blood brain barrier or blood retinal barrier expend about 5 percent more energy maintain the barrier compared to capillary cells elsewhere. This means that healthy capillary cells of the blood brain barrier have 5% more mitochondria on average.

Another group of capillary cells, deep in the brain ventricles, does more secreting into and less pumping out of the cerebrospinal fluid. These capillary cells are known as the *choroid plexus.* The mechanics of pumping and secreting into the CSF by different types of capillary cells results in a specific *blend of bath constituents* whose purpose is to optimize nerve-cell function.

When oxygen delivery is chronically suboptimal relative to brain nerve cell demand, nerve-cell axons and dendrites atrophy, neurotransmitter production diminishes, and there is concomitant loss of connections between other nerve cells both locally and regionally. This causes loss of brain cell mass, which directly corresponds to lost capacity to function. One of the first regions to suffer in the brain from reduced oxygen flow is the long "white matter" axons that retrieve information from the hippocampus to the brain's gray matter. As axons atrophy and connections decrease, the ability to retrieve and learn new information gets compromised. Memory loss is the result. It is often followed by the so called pre-frontal lobe atrophy which is where emotions are regulated and judgements are made regarding the appropriateness of verbal responses, social cues, and the initiation of problem solving.

Brain shrinkage, is directly attributable to dementia as well as a plethora of other neurodegenerative diseases. And it is directly linked to *diffuse vascular inflammatory disease* involving chronic inflammation of the interstitial spaces and basement membranes of all endothelium of the arterial tree from the largest arterial vessels to the smallest capillaries that supply the brain with oxygen. The processes of chronic interstitial space inflammation are induced by chronic seeding of vascular inflammatory free radicals, which directly lead to diffuse arterial basement membrane thickening and obstructive plaque. These combinations stiffen and obstruct arterial blood vessels to the brain to subsequently compromise blood flow, prevent shifts in regional blood flow, and serve notice to the blood brain barrier and brain nerve cells upstream that there will be oxygen deficits that will lead to their atrophy and death (see figure 18 in the appendix).

The process of chronic vascular inflammatory free radical seeding which leads to basement membrane thickening and large vessel obstructive plaque involves blocking the endothelial and capillary cell pivot and swing dances, which enable the emergence of chronic inflammatory momentum and anti-organ. In terms of the brain, the anti-organ will prefer the ischemic-hypoxic and thrombosis card as blocked oxygen delivery creates the most hurt to brain cells. Once brain cells atrophy and die from lack of oxygen it will use scar and amyloid deposits to further suffocate them.

In the discussion about brain health and blood flow to it, one point deserves clarity. Brain metabolism, and the volume of oxygenated blood the brain requires, *remains constant* no matter what human activity is occurring. One liter of blood flow per minute to the brain is required whether the brain is sleeping, r engaged in rigorous mental exercises or watching television. While there are changes in the *distribution* of blood flow in the brain, depending on what activity is being carried out, the *total volume* of flow to the brain does not change. Regional blood-flow shifts occur seamlessly in healthy brains and are brought about by different moods, cognitive behaviors, exercise, and/or sleep. Brain function deteriorates to the extent that that total blood flow falls below one liter per minute and regional blood flow shifting becomes limited or voided by stiff non -responsive chronically inflamed blood vessels.

The implication of this discussion is that the progressive blockage of blood flow to the brain and the inability of the brain's vasculature to shift blood flow to areas of increasing demand, produce a progressive diminution of cognition culminating in what we recognize as dementia. Dementia thereby becomes a spectrum of declining cognition based on whether the brain gets the oxygen it needs or wants. Without the chronic festering of vascular inflammatory free radicals, blood flow to the brain diminishes as endothelial and capillary cell are blocked from dancing. Dementia becomes a natural and predictable outcome.

It is hypothesized that dementia results from a blocked endothelial and capillary cell dance within the vasculature supplying the brain. It involves chronic interstitial space inflammation caused by the persistent festering of vascular inflammatory free radicals and is associated with:

- A chronic expansion of an immune arsenal response to vascular inflammatory free radicals on large vessel endothelial cell basement membranes but also involving capillary cells.

- Perpetuated endothelial and capillary cell outer membrane increases in permeability which requires a sustained flow of energy from mitochondria for active transport of immune arsenal from blood plasma to interstitial spaces and basement membranes to meet the vascular free radical challenge.
- The endothelial and capillary cell dance is blocked and nitric oxide combustion decreases substantially. This blocks among other things capillary and endothelial cell rejuvenation which becomes the mechanism that the chronic inflammatory matrix utilizes to destroy capillary cell homeostasis. Eventually mitochondria die off from irrevocably damaged and incompetent DNA caused from superoxide attachments. As mitochondrial volumes diminish, outer membrane pseudocapillarize surface receptors, pores and voltage gradients. This enables a free- reign to the interstitial space of immune arsenal, which have now pirated the capillary and endothelial cell outer membranes based on orders from the emerged proinflammatory anti-organ.
- Endothelial and capillary cells become a zombied shell and lose their stem and pacing rejuvenation relationship with astrocytes, pericytes, and perhaps, even brain nerve cells.
- As capillary and endothelial cell outer membrane hijacking continues, the immune arsenal arriving from blood plasma is increasingly mismatched to either the large arterial vessel or brain's interstitial space.
- As mismatching continues and immune miscues within the interstitial spaces of either endothelial or capillary cell mount, the emerging anti-organ creates a symbiotic axis with all of the capillary and brain nerve cell partners. Immune arsenal, astrocytes and pericytes switch sides and begin to work for the anti-organ and against the endothelial, capillary and brain cells.
- The proinflammatory momentum garnered by the switch sways the interstitial space in favor of the anti-organ. Astrocytes and pericytes within the blood brain barrier are called upon to produce scar tissue and secrete amyloid, and tau, as blood

flows to nerve cells in the brain decrease. Brain cells suffocate, atrophy and die as amyloid and tau replace them.

- Clinical symptoms become obvious and include fatigue, memory, gate and cognitive loss.
- The full blown effects of chronic inflammation from anti-organ venues expand to include thrombosis (strokes, transient ischemic attacks), seizures, infections (meningitis and encephalitis), movement disorders (Parkinson Syndrome), autoimmune diseases (multiple sclerosis), and brain cancer (meningiomas, astrocytomas, gliomas). The anti-organ will use preexisting genetic vulnerabilities within the brain, in combination with thewhat vascular inflammatory free radicals it has at its disposal, in determining which venue to pursue. Many of these outcomes take advantage of pre -existing genetic influences built into brain cells.

How the Block These Ignoble Outcomes

The worst part of these outcomes is not the fatigue or even the pain, but rather how they rob an individual of the essence and independence. In this sense, brain incarceration from chronic inflammation becomes the most inhumane of abuses that occurs from anti-organ venues. Reversing inflammatory momentum is never easy and certainly does not occur over night. There are no quick fixes but there are solutions when patience and persistence is applied. At least the speed of progression in cognitive decline can be slowed in most instances.

The answer involves a sharp reduction in *all* vascular inflammatory free radicals. Simply stated, the interstitial spaces of endothelial and capillary cells that affront brain cells must be tamed and sanitized. To block further brain cell torture, eliminating a preponderance of vascular inflammatory free radicals gives endothelial and capillary cells the chance to rein in anti-organ influences, as it utilizes free radicals as fuel for its agendas. It does this within interstitial spaces including those of the brain through the persistent recruitment of immune arsenal from the blood plasma. It fuels its venues through misguided immune arsenal,

47

glial and pericyte cells within the interstitial space. What better way to do so than to utilize a steady stream of inflammatory free radicals. By reducing free radicals, the fuel source for chronic inflammation is reduced meaning that there is no impetus for immune arsenal to enter the interstitial space. As their momentum and flow into the space diminish, the door is cracked open for capillary and endothelial cell outer membranes, even in their compromised state, to down shift permeability to then swing mitochondrial combustion to nitric oxide.

This begins a momentum shift within the interstitial space that begins to work for the endothelial, capillary and end organ cells and against the anti-organ. With persistence, the tide turns, as immune arsenal begin to exit the interstitial space, and astrocyte and pericytes start responding again to capillary cells. For their part and because of more nitric oxide combustion, capillary cells have begun to rejuvenate outer membrane receptors, mitochondria and infrastructure and have begun to transmit those rejuvenating signals back to their mesenchymal brethren and to the distressed and isolated brain nerve cells. As these relationship mend, the anti-organ must increasingly find refuge in dark recesses or caverns within the interstitial space produced from previous scarring. Without the immune arsenal, glial and pericytes to help its cause, the anti-organ becomes impotent to implement its venues. It goes into its own solitary confinement, potentially readying itself for the next onslaught of vascular inflammatory free radicals. In this sense the interstitial space becomes a pitch battle of control between the endothelial-capillary cell and the anti-organ. The winner is based on how many and for how long vascular inflammatory free radicals menace the interstitial space.

The hoedown to block anti-organ venues within the brain and elsewhere starts with diet, builds additional momentum with regular exercise, and is further refined through implementing strategies to reduce stress and improve sleep hygiene. Sugar is absolutely toxic to the brain and all sugars must be aggressively reduced for the brain to have any chance of recovery. As has been previously discussed, sugar is rampant in the western diet, comes in many varieties that are not necessarily sweet, and leads to a variety of different vascular inflammatory free radicals that inflame interstitial spaces. Sugars are murky and underreported in food packaging. In addition to sugar, red and processed meats, trans and animal fats must be reduced as they too can menace interstitial spaces.

In addition to sugars, smoking and its 16 or more toxic vascular free radicals that invade the blood stream with every puff wreak havoc on the brain and its surrounding vascular endothelium. Smoking aggressively disrupts endothelial and capillary cell homeostasis and blocks its pivot and swing dance, thereby pushing chronic inflammatory agendas quickly. The brain, heart and lungs are favorite targets, but every end organ can become involved.

If smoking or eating large volumes of sugar persist for 20 years, memory loss begins and forms the basis for early *white matter ischemic changes* seen in the brain. These changes block connections between the brain thinking centers (gray matter) and its information retrieval centers (hippocampus) thereby making learning new information difficult. With progression, the gray matter begins to atrophy in the frontal section of the brain leading to the insidious development of anger, judgement and problem solving deficits.

This same equation of 20 years of exposure to the development of obvious cognitive deficits can also be seen from chronic drug abuse, moderate to heavy alcohol use (more than 14 units of alcohol consumed weekly), or chronic sleep deprivation (less than 6 hours of sleep nightly). The same holds true for medical conditions known to plume chronic interstitial space inflammation, such as such as uncontrolled or poorly controlled diabetes, hypertension and elevated blood plasma LDL cholesterol and triglycerides. When these vascular inflammatory free radical risks are coupled, the risk for dementia escalates even faster. When coupled with advanced age and added inflammatory risk to dementia takes on logarithmic proportions.

The assault against preventing dementia requires a multifactorial approach against all vascular inflammatory risks. In addition to lifestyle adjustments and taming diabetes, hypertension and LDL cholesterol, blood thinning with aspirin or other thinners is recommended as well as an understanding that antioxidant and vitamin supplements are required with advanced age due to evolving deficiency states. The goal is to get endothelia to resume and continue dancing. Doing so stalls out dementia, just like not doing so, brings it on.

Sexual Inadequacy

The capacity for a man or woman to respond sexually to enable a climax, or orgasm, is dependent on a surge of endothelial and capillary cell mitochondrial nitric oxide production. The volume of the surge is based on the health and volume of mitochondria within the capillary cell. The surge causes a large buildup of blood flowing to the penis and clitoris causing these organs to enlarge and stiffen. The enlarged and erect end organs now have more surface area exposed, which through recurring friction, induces peripheral nerve stimulation that eventually leads to involuntary smooth muscle contractions from within the clitoris and penis. These contractions release semen from the penis while readying the uterus to receive them. It also induces intense pleasure and is known as climax.

Successful sexual orgasm brings many different end organs into play but the capacity of the penis and clitoris to enlarge and respond to friction is dependent on capillary cell nitric oxide production. Thus the capacity to have an erection and climax is based on the same mechanics that enable the brain, heart and skeletal muscle to perform well, the capillary cell dance. If downstream large vessel endothelia and upstream capillary cells within the clitoris and penis are dancing, mitochondrial volumes are being maintained and erections to climax will occur. Erectile dysfunction is essentially a disorder of critically reduced mitochondrial volumes in the arteries and capillaries of the penis and clitoris.

Figure 17 in the appendix demonstrates the most important way nitric oxide is produced in capillary mitochondria. In the mitochondrial matrix, *L-arginine,* an essential amino acid, in the presence of oxygen and *activated nitric oxide synthetase,* is converted to *N-hydroxy-L-arginine,* an unstable intermediate. This conversion requires the *cofactor nicotinamide adenine dinucleotide phosphate* (NADPH), which is produced from niacin (vitamin B$_3$). In the presence of oxygen, *L-citrulline* and nitric oxide gas are split off from the unstable intermediate. L-citrulline can be recycled to make more nitric oxide. For nitric oxide combustion to occur, capillary cell mitochondria must not be preoccupied with energy combustion, which as has been discussed, would imply chronic inflammation within interstitial spaces. If chronically preoccupied, mitochondrial volumes diminish and erectile dysfunction occurs.

Therefore, chronic interstitial-space inflammation within the penis and clitoris, which is directly linked to vascular inflammatory free radical seeding, becomes the primary trigger of erectile dysfunction.

Triggering orgasm in both men and women requires input from a variety of peripheral nerves and organs, as well as major input from the brain. All of these end organs are disrupted by chronic inflammation within interstitial spaces. Therefor obtaining successful orgasm involves a coordinated effort that can go awry at many different levels, all of which can be disrupted by chronic interstitial space free radical seeding.

Thus the impact of chronic interstitial space inflammation dwarfs capillary mitochondrial nitric oxide production *everywhere,* to include arteries and capillaries of the penis and clitoris smooth muscle as well as their peripheral nerves and involved end organs. The list is long of the end organs linked to climax but include prostate gland, testicles, ovaries, fallopian tubes, uterus, peripheral nervous system, skeletal muscle, heart, lungs and brain. Without intentional anti-inflammatory interventions, the entire sexual response is blunted at many different levels. Because of so many end organ interconnections that are required in the performance of sex to arousal and orgasm, in older adults, sexual climax becomes a sensitive measuring stick (pardon the pun) as to *how well* chronic interstitial space inflammation has been tamed.

It would stand to reason that a satisfying sex life is a proxy to capillary-cell health and would litmus a pass or fail to chronic inflammatory interstitial space inflammatory control.

Thus the comprehensive blocking interstitial-space and capillary-cell basement-membrane access to vascular inflammatory–free radicals with intentional anti-inflammatory lifestyle choices, as well as with medicinals and supplements where appropriate greatly improves the chances for orgasms to occur. It could even cause a reversal of erectile dysfunction. The renaissance the capillary cell pivot and pendulum swing dance, becomes a safer and far less expensive strategy to resurrect sexual capacity compared to other options, where risks to health usually exceed benefits.

Heart Failure

The force, rate, and duration (length of time) of a heart-muscle cell's capacity to contract depends on how much on demand oxygenated blood can flow to it. It also is dependent on the tone and thickness of the sliding heart actin-myosin muscle filaments. The former is dependent on how much blood flow (oxygen) the capillary cells can actually supply to heart muscle, and the ladder, on the heart muscle filament thickness and volume of mitochondria within individual heart muscle cells. When heart muscle is exercised regularly, both capillary and heart muscle cells perform their respective functions better, with the capillary cells pacing the improvement.

The capacity to deliver large volumes of blood to hardworking heart muscle becomes dependent on how well large vessel coronary endothelium and upstream capillary cell mitochondria can increase nitric oxide combustion. The response is two-fold and interdependent on both the large arterial coronary arteries are that are supplying blood (and oxygen) and the upstream capillaries receiving the blood on the basis of what and how they signal. If lumens are obstructed from basement membrane plaque buildup as a result of chronic inflammation, no matter what upstream capillary message is, the blood flow response will be less than desired. This means there is *disconnect* between what the heart muscle needs and what it gets. This does not bode well for heart muscle in the long term.

Larger coronary arteries aside, the capacity of capillary cell mitochondria to expand nitric oxide production to increase on demand blood flow (oxygen) to heart muscle is dependent on the volume of mitochondria they have within their cell. Mitochondrial volumes become dependent on whether there has been successful rejuvenation of the capillary cell, which is dependent on their ability to dance, which occurs when interstitial space inflammation has been subdued. With any chronic interstitial space inflammation, capillary cell mitochondrial volumes will be depleted and their capacity to generate nitic oxide in response to on- demand requests from heart muscle for more oxygen will be diminished.

Chronic interstitial space inflammation affects oxygen delivery to heart muscle in at least two ways. First the inflammatory milieu within the interstitial space between capillary and heart muscle cell laden with inflammatory debris and is therefore not conducive to the clean passive diffusion of oxygen gas between the capillary and heart muscle cell. Second, oxygen delivery can be blocked by downstream reductions in blood flow caused by large vessel (coronary artery) obstructive plaque. Both of these conditions, as an expression of chronic interstitial space inflammation, can impair oxygen delivery to heart muscle.

One outcome to this disconnect of oxygen demand to delivery is for capillary cells to scramble and produce growth factors in attempts to make new capillaries to theoretically bring more blood flow. Sometimes this scrambling can help, particularly if there is sufficient *collateral circulation* from other large coronary arteries that can compensate for lost blood flow from the obstructed coronary. Their growth factor scrambling will fall on deaf ears however, if there is no such coronary artery collateral easement.

When capillary cells run out of options to increase blood flow and oxygen delivery to heart muscle, hypoxic- ischemic events occur and are known as angina. Angina can cause chest pain, fatigue or shortness of breath. If ignored it can lead to a *heart attack myocardial infarction) or even sudden death.* When heart muscle dies from a heart attack and the heart survives the attack, the dead muscle is replaced by scar tissue which increases risk for *heart failure, valve leakages and sudden death from a malignant arrhythmia.* Heart failure causes increased fatigue and breathlessness with exertion and can severely lessen activity. All of these outcomes can be attributable to a persistently blocked endothelial and capillary cell dance caused by chronic inflammation and the subsequent venues within the interstitial space implemented by the anti-organ. In this case, as it so often does in end organs that are very oxygen sensitive, it involves thrombosis and the development of scar tissue. How the anti-organ facilitates thrombosis through the genesis of progressive larger vessel coronary artery obstructive plaque leading heart attack and heart failure is depicted in figure 18 in the appendix.

With so much at stake on the wellness-prevention side to the heart and brain equation, you would think the medical industrial complex would be more interested. Instead it remains fixed on *disease treatment models*, which require expensive drugs and technology to treat with increasingly narrow therapeutic benefits. It is so not the future to taming health care expenses while enabling good health practices. Simply stated, disease treatment is a very expensive, often requires sophisticated surveillance, is wrought with complications and self -perpetuates plumes of more and expensive interventions. The disease treatment model has never been more obvious than what is has become in cardiology. None of these interventions that involve stents, bypass grafts, pacing systems, defibrillators, or imaging procedures produce long lasting results unless the elephant in the room is addressed, *vascular inflammatory free radicals.* Those reductions, in contrast to disease treatments, can be done at home, an involve adjustments in behavioral mechanics and perhaps some inexpensive medicinals or supplements.

All of these aforementioned forays into cardiology disease treatment through the medical-industrial complex, do save lives and in most instances are well intentioned, but also pace on drag on well- being from side effects, required surveillance, and the risk of interventional failures. Worries accumulate that in themselves reduce quality of life. We often can't identify what the next pain, breathlessness or fatigue is caused from and so we often stress or lose sleep from the anxiety it causes. In this manner, the increase in stress hormones and the inflammation they cause to our interstitial spaces caused from anxiety, can exceed the benefits of all the different interventions. Without a master plan involving chronic inflammatory prevention and wellness, being a chronic heart, lung, liver, joint, kidney or brain patient, becomes a joyless and often anxiety provoking experience of appointments, endless procedures and expensive interventions.

As might be expected, chronic inflammation that is associated with heart disease is also a systemic one that involves at some level all other end organs. In addition, the effects of heart disease can adversely affect all other end organs by limiting blood flow and oxygen delivery to them. So chronic inflammation is not isolated to one place or space, but ties together the entire endothelial and capillary arterial system as well as all the end organs they attend to. As chronic inflammation takes over the interstitial spaces of end organs, and as capillary cells throughout the arterial tree stop dancing, end organs fail often in tandem. Fatigue, pain and aging materialize exponentially as they fail. In a sense, this can be described as *metastatic chronic inflammation* of the interstitial spaces.

Sarcopenia

The anti-aging of skeletal muscle is reflected in its capacity to perform intensive and sustained contractions and then recover quickly to do it all over again. Similar to heart muscle, *well-toned* skeletal-muscle cells have high concentrations of mitochondria abutting their outer membranes (*sarcolemma*). When the sliding actin-myosin filaments are thick and dense, skeletal-muscle *mass* is increased, which increases their potential force of contraction. Figure 27 in the appendix demonstrates a cross section of a skeletal-muscle cell. The cell is surrounded by a sarcolemma (outer membranes), which borders the interstitial space adjacent to their partners the capillary cells. Skeletal-muscle mitochondria lie close to the sarcolemma to have immediate access to oxygen, glucose, and fatty acids arriving through capillary cells. They utilize these raw materials to make large volumes of energy, particularly when skeletal-muscle actin-myosin filament sliding (skeletal-muscle contraction) is robust. The volume of oxygen and energy substrate received and the amount of energy (and calcium ion release) produced by skeletal-muscle mitochondria, coupled with the thickness and density of their actin-myosin filaments, determines the rate, force, and duration of skeletal-muscle contraction.

For skeletal-muscle cells to perform optimally, they must have the following:

- a sufficient volume of on- demand blood containing oxygen and energy substrate
- a sufficient volume of mitochondria to support actin-myosin sliding (muscle contraction)
- a sufficient density and thickness of actin-myosin filaments
- absence of chronic interstitial space inflammation

All these pieces are important, but the last one becomes the predictor of the other three. If the interstitial space is chronically inflamed, it predicts declining skeletal-muscle function. As has been a repeating mantra, as chronic interstitial space inflammation progresses, it reduces the efficient exchange of oxygen and energy substrate between the capillary and skeletal muscle. It also causes capillary-cell outer membranes to become preoccupied with pushing immune arsenal into the interstitial space which blocks their swing dance to nitric oxide production form their mitochondria. When the capillary cell dance is blocked, rejuvenation does not occur and their mitochondrial volumes decrease, leading to pseudocapilarization of outer membranes and then blocked stemming and pacing of critical rejuvenating feedback loops to its interstitial space partners and end organ. The causes a coalescence of the chronic inflammatory matrix which sets a proinflammatory agenda within the interstitial space that targets capillary cell outer membranes permeability, immune arsenal and mesenchymal cells. Once the agenda is established, the anti-organ can emerge which begins processes of creating destructive venues to the end organ. In skeletal muscle these venues involve thrombosis, hypoxic-ischemic events, scarring and sarcopenia but can also include infections, cancers and autoimmune complex diseases as well. All of these anti-organ venues are linked to fatigue, pain and aging.

When skeletal muscle tone and mass diminish, less energy substrate will be utilized, regardless of the activity. Duration and intensity or muscle contraction decrease meaning we can't do an activity as much or for as long. As sarcopenia increases and energy substrate utilization decreases, insulin resistance leading to adult diabetes becomes commonplace. Decreased muscle mass and tone create inflammatory momentum that parlays less activity with increasing weight, stiff and painful joints as well as posture and gait problems. In this sense, sarcopenia cascades a set of powerful proinflammatory influences, each of which abets more chronic inflammation. It also suggests the corollary, that maintaining muscle mass and tone from regular exercise could prevent all these abetments and the inflammatory cascades that follow.

Exercised skeletal muscle nicely demonstrates the crisscrossing interplay of feedback loops between capillary and skeletal-muscle mitochondria. As exercised skeletal-muscle mitochondria call out for more oxygen and energy substrate to facilitate a greater rate and force of actin and myosin filament sliding, capillary-cell mitochondria pendulum swing combustion in the *opposite* direction to nitric oxide to increase blood flow (and oxygen/energy substrate) to the skeletal muscle. Exercise therefore supports nitric oxide driven rejuvenation of capillary-cell infrastructure, mitochondrial volumes, outer-membrane receptors, and nuclear telomeres, while simultaneously facilitating increased skeletal-muscle function. As well toned and exercised skeletal muscle takes on energy substrate like a sponge to water, insulin resistance dramatically reduces, which cascades to reduce blood LDL cholesterol levels and blood pressure. Thus exercise reduces multiple vascular inflammatory risks while also inducing a robust rejuvenation of endothelial and capillary cell mitochondria and infrastructure as they support increased blood flow to skeletal muscle. Because of all these add-ons, exercise reduces chronic inflammation everywhere.

When skeletal muscle exercise is completed, their mitochondria crisscross combustion again with their capillary cell mitochondrial brethren. In this phase, skeletal-muscle mitochondria pendulum swing combustion to nitric oxide as they rejuvenate their infrastructure, while capillary mitochondria shift combustion towards energy, to assist in the clean-up process of removing waste residues from the interstitial space. All of this cum bay yah homeostasis is optimal as long as chronic inflammation is not festering in the interstitial space.

So, capillary cells pace a well- coordinated skeletal-muscle and capillary-cell crisscrossing mitochondrial combustion relationship which is tied into capillary cell outer membrane permeability and the pivot and swing dance. The potent anti-inflammatory momentum, linked to regular exercise, reduces risks for sarcopenia as well as all the vascular inflammatory free radicals tied to insulin resistance and adult diabetes. Skeletal muscles were intended to be used regularly.

Aging: The Emergence of Multi-Organ Chronic Inflammation and Failure

Proinflammatory lifestyle choices do not occur in a vacuum and without consequences. The pattern of accumulating chronic interstitial-space inflammation from the pestering of vascular inflammatory free-radicals interrupts the capillary cell dance thereby perpetuating additional chronic inflammation. Multi organ compromises occur, serious chronic and life threatening illnesses result, and debilitating fatigue and pain become universal symptoms connected to chronic inflammation.

Blocking the capillary cell dance is the gateway as to how chronic inflammation establishes a foothold within interstitial spaces. Once established, it begins the process of disassembling all of the pieces within the interstitial space to conform to its emerging purpose. It does so by confusing the purpose of interstitial space immune arsenal and mesenchymal cells. The result is to create a more random and ineffective immune chaos, inflammatory chaos if you will. This creates ideal interstitial space conditions that coalesce to form the proinflammatory interstitial space matrix. With the matrix in place, chronic inflammation can extend its reach with a primary objective being to pirate control of capillary cell outer membrane permeability. The message and the immune response that it invokes perpetuates even more interstitial space inflammatory chaos.

What is central to the inflammatory matrix agenda is the use of immune arsenal that was intended for use by the capillary cell for its own purpose. This switch in interstitial space alignment, coupled with persistent vascular free radical seeding, forms the basis for developing unstoppable inflammatory momentum and the hijacking of the capillary cell outer membranes.

At some level of inflammatory chaos, the gloves come off and the proinflammatory tilt within the interstitial space shift momentum to favor riding the wave of chronic inflammatory influences. Once the capillary cell outer membranes have been hijacked the coast has been cleared for the emergence of the anti-organ. The anti-organ differs from the matrix in that it has the power to organize venues within the interstitial that are a direct affront to the integrity of the capillary-end organ relationship. The venues, either separately or in aggregate, lead the interstitial space to an Armageddon experience that culminates in anyone of a series of chronic or life threatening illnesses linked to waves of fatigue and pain. Their debilitating effects metastasize to other endothelia and end organs as a new systemic homeostasis is formed that ages and distorts health in all end organs rather than promote it.

Taking advantage of every cue, even taking into account a given end organ's unique genetic vulnerability, the anti-organ will turn over every mechanism at its disposal to use against the end organ. It begins with chronic vascular free radicals seeding of the interstitial space, which spreads to block the capillary cell pivot and swing dance. It culminates in the unleashing of an array of different interstitials pace venues designed to hurt, even kill the end organ. The anti-organ will take what it can and when it can and use it against the end organ.

A fallacy of disease treatment models is that we put the cart before the horse. By ignoring the root cause of chronic inflammation, and instead focus on the effect, we treat outcomes. Doing so perpetuates more adverse outcomes and complications from treatments which spirals treatment for more adverse outcomes and complications from treatment. Disease treatment self -perpetuates itself similar to how chronic inflammation within interstitial spaces does the same.

Disease treatment is one more mechanism the anti-organ can utilize to spiral next level interstitial space venues that work against the end organ and its homeostasis. Treatments of cancer or infections create resistance and superinfections. Trying to reverse scar tissue in the brain, such as amyloid deposition, backfires to create empty space without addressing why it formed in the first place. Treating autoimmune complex disease with modern chemotherapy often leads to lymphomas or the development of bone cancers.

This is not to say that disease treatment is not well intentioned and can stop the course of serious illnesses and even save lives. In balance disease treatment truly works in emergencies but let's not confuse acuity with chronic inflammation. In the longer run of our daily lives, disease treatment is short sighted and misses the point. Given the new understanding about chronic inflammation and how it disseminates it is time to welcome a wellness model of prevention, which is more cost effective, addresses root causes of chronic inflammation, and is better suited for making adjustments in daily living. The time is upon us where we can no longer ignore the basis for why we become ill and expect a shot, surgery or drug to cure us, and then move on and do the same stupid things.

When we choose the band aide over the root cause we enable the anti-organ effect. Simply stated, the intent of disease treatment is to treat disease. Occasionally disease treatment stumbles into chronic inflammatory treatment, but it is not by intent. As we move deeper into the twenty-first century, the charade of more expensive tech, drugs and invasive interventions must be replaced with a more natural and common sense approach to health. Manipulating genes to treat disease is a good business model but is self –serving, as it does little to stem bad habits or halt chronic inflammation Let's turn the page before our health care system goes broke.

Pain, Fatigue, and Aging: A Fait Accompli?

What becomes clear in discussing the demise of endothelia and the capillary-cell is that chronic inflammation is fueled by vascular inflammatory free radical seeds. Chronic inflammation then has the ability within the interstitial space to go undercover and begin manipulating the mechanics of interstitial space homeostasis, to eventually utilize them for its own purpose. As it does, it brings together pieces within the interstitial space, originally used by the capillary cell for interstitial space sanitation, to its own benefit by conforming them to a new identity. The newly minted coalition of outed immune arsenal, mesenchymal cells and inflammatory debris becomes a matrix, whose agenda is to continue extorting the interstitial space to favor chronic inflammation. With each turn of momentum, chronic inflammation increases its scope and stranglehold in the battle for control of the interstitial space.

Blocking the influx of vascular inflammatory free radicals into the interstitial space blocks the feeding reservoir of chronic inflammation. The foundation for this reversal is to starve chronic inflammation, reverse the momentum to mobilize more immune arsenal into the interstitial space from blood plasma, thereby enabling an already compromised endothelial and capillary cell the opportunity to downshift its outer membrane permeability. The door opens for resumption of the capillary cell pivot and swing dance. As the rust comes off and as mitochondria swing combustion to nitric oxide, the capillary cell stands half a chance to get back its own integrity.

Starving chronic interstitial space inflammation requires lifestyle adjustments more than anything else. Without a lifestyle about face, inflammatory momentum wins no matter how much disease treatment intervention we spend money on.

Aging becomes a reflection of how much chronic inflammation has accumulated in our interstitial spaces. Reversing chronic inflammation with a lifestyle overhaul is the basis for wellness. It not only addresses the root cause of inflammation, it also reverses *aging signs and symptoms*, such as fatigue and pain. By restoring interstitial space sanitation, while also stemming and pacing rejuvenation, the capillary cell dance makes end organs function better and last longer, as it pushes residuals of the anti-organ into isolation. It's possible, that lifestyle could even push adverse gene reversals. Making better choices about how we eat, drink, breathe, move, and sleep produces its own sets of anti-inflammatory momentum that cascade benefits to even cause chromosomes to heal.

Enabling the endothelial-capillary cell dance blocks the "fait accompli." End organs don't have to fail with age. Instead, getting older can be much grander, to expand on rather than contract its repertoire of collective experience. We think better, move quicker for much longer periods in life, perhaps decades longer. Age does not have to mean I'm done. Personal relevance increases rather than sets with the sun.

Changing the course of chronic inflammation really means what it implies. It requires a different mindset from the moment we open our eyes in the morning from sleep. It invokes an intentional set of priorities and activity levels. We move away from *addictive and reactionary* activities that control our minds, time and block our senses. Instead we move towards being more *intentional* about choice, to nurture a different mindset such as taking a walk in nature, engaging in yoga or breathing exercises, cultivating a garden, or finding quiet time to read a book, engage in music or enjoy a pleasant conversation. It is about finding a pace of life that is not overbearing while also providing opportunity to quiet the mind in preparation for uninterrupted sleep. We become intentionally gentle about how we treat that which encompasses our essence.

When the lifestyle page is turned, we become more *intuitive* about how to make the right choices. Timing and judgement improve regarding what to eat, how to exercise and how to pace the day. If the context yields combinations of contentment, joy and peace we are winning the war against chronic inflammation.

Welcome home to a new beginning.

Chapter 3

CAPILLARY-CELL MITOCHONDRIA: MORE THAN A MOTOR

It is now evident that the capillary-cell dance forms the basis for preventing illness and improving end-organ performance. This requires lifestyle readjustments to reduce chronic inflammatory free radical influences in the interstitial spaces of end organs. The cornerstone mechanics of the capillary cell dance involves outer membrane permeability but the execution of permeability goes through mitochondrial combustion.

Mitochondria found throughout the body all have similar anatomy and physiology. In contrast to capillary cells, which utilize anaerobic mechanisms within their cytoplasm for 90% of their energy, end-organ energy production is almost completely dependent on mitochondria. In the case of the heart and brain, it can be upwards of 90-95%. The generation of that percentage of end organ energy by mitochondria requires on demand infusions of oxygen and energy substrate. This translates into sudden and sometimes dramatic increases in blood volumes (and hence more oxygen and energy substrate delivery) to end organs. This fluctuation of blood volumes to needy end organs requires an effective capillary cell dance and a robust production of nitric oxide from their mitochondria.

As an example, when heart muscle cells are called upon to contract faster and with more force to move more blood through its four chambers, *all* of the energy required to uptick work capacity comes from *mitochondrial combustion*. In contrast, while heart muscle mitochondria are cranking energy combustion to increase the rate and force of actin-myosin sliding, capillary cell mitochondrial are doing the opposite. Instead, they have downshifted energy production and have swung combustion to nitric oxide to facilitate increases in blood flow (oxygen and energy substrate) to the har working heart muscle. Conversely, when the heart muscle cell actin-myosin sliding slows down, their mitochondria don't need as much oxygen to produce as much energy.

Instead, as they swing combustion to nitric oxide to rejuvenate their infrastructure, the capillary cell mitochondria swing and pace combustion in the opposite direction, towards energy. Dong so provides capillary cell outer membranes with energy to be used in active transport of immune arsenal and other venues that provide necessary sanitation and clean- up of the interstitial space that is required after the heart muscle's hard work. The cleanup guarantees quality assurance of optimal interstitial space homeostasis, such that when heart muscle cells fires back up again to require large influxes of oxygen or energy substrate, it is generously supplied by capillary cells through the interstitial space in seamless fashion. In this manner, the health of the capillary cell, sanitation of the interstitial space, and the capacity of heart muscle cells to function optimally are all based on how well capillary cell outer membranes and mitochondria are dancing the pivot and swing.

Competent capillary cell outer membrane flux in permeability is codependent on how effective mitochondrial combustion responds to it and visa-versa. Capillary cell fluxing stems and paces the pulsing of different feedback loops within the interstitial space that defines intent. This is to say pulsed capillary cell feedback loops maintain interstitial space sanitation, coordinated through mesenchymal cells and immune arsenal, provide oxygen and nutrient for optimal end organ function, while rejuvenating itself and its mesenchymal and end organ partners. Each purpose that induces capillary cell fluxing in one direction reflexively feeds back to also supports benefits in the other direction. This allows capillary cells to be multi purposed.

By pulsing immune surveillance of the interstitial space, it is implied that small amounts of containable inflammation serve a purpose towards optimal homeostasis. That is, small amounts of contaminant or vascular inflammatory free radicals residing within the interstitial space could actually improve capillary cell health, whereas larger amounts don't as they can fester and lead to chronic inflammation.

Therein lies the capillary and endothelial cell permeability rub. It is likely that with the passage of time, the volume of acceptable free radical infringement within the interstitial space is a moving target with the bias trending to lower levels being acceptable. This would mean that for the interstitial space to remain optimally sanitized with aging, vascular inflammatory free radical penetration must be biased towards further reduction.

How did capillary cells generally, and mitochondria specifically, become responsible for so much arbitrage? Let's probe mitochondrial mechanics, to find out.

Anatomy and Physiology of Mitochondria

Figure 1 in the appendix demonstrates the anatomy and physiology of a mitochondria.

Mitochondria are intracellular *organelles* that have similar properties comparable to bacteria. While mitochondrial shape does not change much from human cell to cell, their size and volumes (mass) within a given cell do. Mitochondria are comprised of an inner membrane, an outer membrane, an intermembrane space, and a core matrix. Together, the matrix and inner membrane form their core infrastructure that enables the combustion of energy (ATP) and nitric oxide. The mitochondrial matrix also provides the necessary mechanics that facilitates a potent inner-membrane voltage gradient, store calcium, manufacture heme, as well as produce antioxidants, proteins and other enzymes. It utilizes its combustion apparatus to establish powerful feedback loops with outer membranes, other organelles, the nucleus, and beyond, to even include other cellular partners outside of and within the interstitial space.

A key element to mitochondrial success in producing energy is the inner-membrane clumping of five *cytochrome* complexes. The cytochrome chambers facilitate the transfer of electrons (see appendix, figure 2). By doing so, hydrogen atoms are split off and released into the intermembrane space. This creates a radical divergence of hydrogen between the mitochondrial matrix and intermembrane space, which enables the high-voltage electric current of the inner membrane. This very potent *electric gradient* is what allows the mitochondria to tightly regulate the movement of hydrogen, magnesium, calcium, and energy in and out of their matrix. It also assists in providing a pace to the metabolism of pyruvate, fatty acids, and heme. It becomes integral in energy production as hydrogen is reintroduced to the mitochondrial matrix through cytochrome V to facilitate the conversion of ADP to ATP. Finally, it serves as the basis for feedback loop adjustment in mitochondrial combustion between energy and nitric oxide.

A key element in this feedback loop adjustment from energy to nitric oxide is activation within the mitochondrial matrix of nitric oxide synthetase. When activated it blocks cytochrome electron transfer (thereby blocking energy combustion), while at the same time facilitating the use of oxygen to produce nitric oxide gas. Activation of nitric oxide synthetase is based on feedback loops generated by a downshift in capillary cell outer membrane permeability. The downward shift in outer membrane permeability is brought about by less demand for energy. As a result, unused ATP and calcium ions accumulate in capillary cell cytoplasm, which then feeds back to the mitochondrial matrix to stop energy combustion and activate nitric oxide synthetase. In this manner, capillary and endothelial cell mitochondria swing their combustion back and forth from energy to nitric oxide based on how much energy, and calcium ions are feeding back to it at any given moment. If there is less energy and calcium the capillary cell's cytoplasm, the inference to mitochondrial is to swing combustion towards energy and release more calcium and visa-versa. The link to these feedback loops is nitric oxide synthetase and whether it is activated or not.

In addition to facilitating energy and nitric oxide combustion, the mitochondrial matrix houses infrastructure that facilitates the mobilization of hydrogen to the cytochromes, the storage of calcium, and the production of acetyl coenzyme A, heme and antioxidants. Acetyl coenzyme A is produced from energy substrates primarily derived from *pyruvate* and *fatty acids* (see appendix, figures 3 and 5). Acetyl CoA, becomes the *hub of combustion*, as it can enter the *Krebs cycle* (see appendix, figure 4) to facilitate hydrogen transfer to the cytochromes for energy production, or it can be shuttled to *ribosomes and smooth endoplasmic reticulum* outside of the mitochondria to be used for protein synthesis, repair and replacement. The former facilitates outer membrane active transport whereas the ladder forms the basis for capillary cell rejuvenation of outer membrane receptors, mitochondria and infrastructure.

Other proteins and enzymes within the matrix are utilized in manufacturing heme from iron (see appendix, figure 14), facilitate the storage and movement of magnesium and calcium ions, and restore depleted antioxidants. Some of these proteins are coded for my mitochondrial DNA, which unlike nuclear chromosomal DNA, lacks a protective telomere cap. Because mitochondrial DNA is naked and resides near the combustion apparatus in the mitochondrial matrix, it is vulnerable to cross linkage from lingering free radicals such as superoxide.

The risk for superoxide mitochondrial DNA damage is an important reason why capillary mitochondrial combustion *must* pendulum swing back and forth. Doing so avoids superoxide free radical lingering that occurs from excessive combustion of energy. Pendulum swinging combustion also helps to restock antioxidants as combustion shifting reduces antioxidant utilization by generating less of one type of free radical. That is, combusting energy and nitric oxide results in different kinds of free radicals exhaust. As one free radical exhaust is formed from say nitric oxide combustion, the antioxidant to the free radical not produced will increase and visa-versa. Thus swinging combustion ensures re accumulation of antioxidants while also reducing the risk for over utilization. Without pendulum swinging combustion free radicals linger, antioxidants become exhausted, DNA damage escalates, protein synthesis when it occurs is defective and mitochondrial volumes diminish precipitously.

Figure 2 in the appendix summarizes how the mitochondrial inner-membrane cytochromes *push-out* (cytochromes I–IV) and *pull-in* (cytochrome V) hydrogen ions from the matrix to eventually result in energy production. In the figure cytochromes (I–IV), via electron transfer, pull hydrogen ions from the matrix and subsequently push them (cytochrome V) back into the matrix, where they are utilized by the enzyme ATP synthetase in the presence of ADP, oxygen, and phosphorus to convert ADP to make ATP. While this is going on, capillary cell outer membranes have increased permeability and are utilizing energy for active transport. It is also a time where nitric oxide synthetase activity within the mitochondrial matrix is inactive.

Mitochondrial Energy Substrates

Endothelial and capillary cell mitochondria produce energy (ATP) by combusting oxygen in the presence of ATP synthetase, ADP (adenosine diphosphate), phosphorus, and hydrogen. They utilize energy substrates—pyruvate (from glucose), fatty acids (odd- and even-numbered carbon chains), and in some cases, ketone bodies (specialized energy units made in the liver from fatty acids)—to produce acetyl CoA. Matrix oxidative machinery, including that utilized in the Krebs cycle, facilitates a steady stream of hydrogen ions, which are then transported by FAD and NAD (*flavin-adenine dinucleotide* and *nicotinamide-adenine dinucleotide*) to the cytochromes on the inner membrane.

Energy substrates that are utilized to produce acetyl CoA in endothelial and capillary cell mitochondria usually come from carbohydrates and sugars that are reduced to glucose and then pyruvate, and fatty acids of various lengths. In starvation or very low calorie diets, energy substrate can also come from ketone bodies, which are synthesized in the liver or as a result of protein catabolism. Most cells, including capillary cells, have an elaborate anaerobic (without the use of oxygen) check-and-balance system within their cytoplasm for converting sugar (glucose) to pyruvate (also known as *glycolysis*) or pyruvate back to sugar (known as *gluconeogenesis*) to maintain a steady state pyruvate concentration. Pyruvate concentrations can fluctuate for different reason but generally it is metabolically favorable within the capillary cell for glucose to be converted to pyruvate through glycolysis and then be utilized by mitochondria to produce acetyl CoA. This implies less insulin resistance and better utilization of pyruvate within mitochondria.

When glucose, a *monosaccharide simple sugar,* is converted to pyruvate, it can be transported into the mitochondrial matrix. Once there, with just *one simple enzymatic step,* pyruvate can be quickly converted to acetyl CoA (see appendix, figure 3). If mitochondria are combusting energy, acetyl CoA is shuttled to the Krebs cycle (see appendix, figure 4) to be reduced and then to release hydrogen, which is then transported to the cytochromes to make energy. If mitochondria are combusting nitric oxide, acetyl CoA is mobilized to ribosomes and rough endoplasmic reticulum for protein synthesis. This provides rejuvenation of outer membrane protein receptors and capillary cell infrastructure, but most importantly it resuscitates mitochondrial volumes (see appendix figure 7).

Fatty acids of up to 16 carbons in length can also be shuttled into the mitochondria to make acetyl co A (see appendix, figure 5) through a process known as beta oxidation. Fatty acid conversion to acetyl CoA is less efficient that pyruvate, but releases more hydrogen for more potential energy. It also creates more exhaust creating the risk for more superoxide free radicals. Fatty acid combustion is biased to occur in conditions favoring insulin resistance and diabetes. This means it is utilized in mitochondria in preference to pyruvate for production of acetyl CoA, which then shifts pyruvate in the cytoplasm to be converted to glucose by gluconeogenesis. If this is persistent, not only does glucose increase in the blood stream to worsen diabetes, but increased fatty acid combustion to make acetyl co A potentially increases superoxide free radical exhaust.

With aging, obesity, sarcopenia, and inactivity, fatty acids can gain a competitive advantage over pyruvate in mitochondrial combustion. This subtle shift in fatty acid over pyruvate utilization over time can potentiate more DNA free radical damage and subsequent loss of mitochondrial volumes in all cells, including capillary and endothelial cells.

Inflammatory damage to capillary cell mitochondria and infrastructure doubles down, when fatty acids are utilized in favor of pyruvate in the setting of persistent mitochondrial energy combustion. In diabetes, the mitochondrial preference to fatty acids coupled with increased vascular inflammatory free radical accumulation within interstitial spaces, produces a double whammy proinflammatory effect on capillary and endothelial cells to accelerate their declines. In this setting not only to free radicals aggregate to expand interstitial space inflammation, but inside the capillary cell mitochondria, superoxide accumulates rapidly form the combinations of excessive energy combustion and fatty acid utilization. Elevated superoxide levels become a wrecking-ball to nearby membranes and DNA surfaces, rapidly degrading capillary cell infrastructure, mitochondrial volumes and pseudocapillarizing its outer membranes. It becomes a perfect introduction to the anti-organ.

Beta-Oxidation

Fatty acids are short and long methylated chains of carbon, often branched like a tree, and derived from both animal and plant sources. Fatty acids of up to sixteen carbons in length may enter the mitochondrial matrix as whole molecules. Larger fatty acids must be broken down into a smaller size by liposomes within the cytoplasm before entering mitochondria. Fatty acids that are saturated are more stable in heat or light and have fewer carbons that are double bonded to oxygen. Polyunsaturated fatty acids have carbons with more double bonds and fewer hydrogen attachments, which enables them to twist or bend when heated causing them to reconfigure from a cis to a trans- fat. *Trans -fats*, when incorporated into membrane infrastructure, disrupt membrane function and become proinflammatory. When capillary cell outer membranes are messaged to create receptor exposures, trans-fat integration can cause silent or inappropriate membrane bending thereby nullifying precise or nuanced receptor exposures. This has the effect of compounding capillary cell membrane receptor mistakes resulting in a more random immune arsenal mobilization into the interstitial space. These are the types of cracks that perpetuate chronic inflammation, destabilize the interstitial space, overheat capillary mitochondria, and open the door for an upgraded interstitial a space chronic inflammatory agenda. The momentum of trans-fat assimilation into membrane surfaces undoubtedly increases an accelerated chronic inflammatory risk in interstitial spaces.

In addition to the saturated and unsaturated classification, fatty acids can be subdivided into *long chained* (sixteen to twenty-five carbons) or *short chained* (four carbons or fewer), and can have *odd* (usually from plants) or *even* numbers of carbons. Because of fatty acid variability, beta-oxidation to produce acetyl CoA is more elaborate (see appendix, figure 5), slower, and results in a more diversified end product compared to pyruvate oxidation. Beta-oxidation of *odd-chained* fatty acids, in contrast to *even-chained* fatty acids, yields acetyl CoA and *propionyl CoA*, instead of just pure acetyl CoA. *Propionyl CoA* can then be converted, to *succinyl CoA*, which like acetyl CoA, can also act as a combustion hub with slightly different nuance.

Beta-oxidation of *plant fatty acids* slows the pace and diversifies the final concentration of produced acetyl CoA. Thus, beta-oxidation of long-branched chain monounsaturated plant fatty acids both trickles and diversifies acetyl CoA production. This *trickle-diversity effect* of plant based fatty acid oxidation can help shift the competitive balance of mitochondrial combustion towards pyruvate. The implication is that plant oils—especially when used in small amounts—improve pyruvate utilization, increase glycolysis, and decrease gluconeogenesis. This limits insulin resistance and reduces the proinflammatory effects of elevated blood sugars and advanced glycation end product free radicals.

The Electron Transport Chain (ETC)

The "horse" of mitochondrial energy production is the *electron transport chain* (ETC) and the inner membrane *cytochrome system* (see appendix, figure 2). As previously discussed, the ETC is housed in an elaborate five-compartment cytochrome system within the mitochondrial inner membrane.

How does the electron transport chain work? The ETC is best utilized when cells require a sudden surge of energy production. In the capillary cell, that would occur when their outer membranes require increased mobilization of inflammatory mediators from blood plasma to or from the interstitial space using energy for active transport. The infrastructure within the mitochondrial matrix, including the Krebs cycle, is built to support electron transfer, by breaking down energy substrate, causing the release of hydrogen, and then transporting it to the awaiting cytochromes. It is the dumping of hydrogen into the awaiting cytochromes that fuels electron transfer.

Cytochrome complex I is the first in a series of clumped proteins, cofactors and enzymes that retrieve hydrogen from transporters within the mitochondrial matrix. Within the cytochrome itself, proteins composed of mostly heme rings are utilized to transfer electrons from one cytochrome to the next. As electrons are transferred, hydrogen is released into the intermembrane space thereby creating a disparity of hydrogen from one side of the inner membrane compared to the other. This disparity forms the basis for the potent electromechanical inner membrane gradient.

Electron transfer is accomplished by proteins in cytochromes that contain positively charged binding metals where the electrons attach and release to the next binding metal. Central to and within the mosaic of cytochrome electron transfer is the heme ring and its centrally located iron metal. The heme ring, and its configuration within the cytochrome series of electron transfers, is an important contributor to the mechanics of electron movement and hydrogen release into the intermembrane space. As such heme becomes pivotal to both the hydrogen reservoir in the intermembrane space and the management of the inner membrane voltage gradient.

In all cells, including capillary cells, the production of large volumes of ATP in mitochondria by electron transport becomes the basis for producing quick on-demand surges of energy that are required for both specific and elaborate cellular function as well as supporting feedback loop management and the subsequent sub loop momentum it generates. Simply stated, when mitochondria can make large volumes of energy by combusting oxygen, cells can specialize and do more than they could when they could only use the much slower and cumbersome fermentation or anaerobic metabolism.

When energy is produced by combustion, the mitochondrial matrix also releases calcium ions, which in endothelial and capillary cell, further augments increases in outer membrane permeability of immune arsenal. In end organ cells, the surge of energy production by mitochondrial combustion increases their capacity to perform their specific functions. This surge is dependent on receiving enough oxygen to do so, which then falls back on endothelia and capillary cells to facilitate its delivery by increasing blood flows.

The regulation of the capillary cell pacing of mitochondrial energy and nitric oxide combustion is dependent on permeability fluxing generated from capillary cell outer-membranes. The permeability pivot or lack thereof becomes dependent on how much and how long inflammatory free radicals fester within the interstitial space. When festering is contained, free radical influence in the interstitial space diminishes. As such, immune-arsenal requirements to neutralize then commensurately diminish. The anti-inflammatory affect builds momentum by reducing capillary cell outer membrane active transport energy demands, thereby causing unused ATP and calcium to buildup in the cytoplasm and feedback to mitochondria to stop energy combustion. This activates mitochondrial matrix nitric oxide synthetase which simultaneously blocks electron transfer through the cytochromes while initiating combustion of nitric oxide. With the nitric oxide shift, acetyl CoA is shuttled away from the Krebs cycle and towards ribosomes and smooth endoplasmic reticulum within the cytoplasm to provide impetus for protein synthesis. This shift in acetyl CoA purpose from providing hydrogen ions for energy combustion to facilitating protein synthesis becomes the feedback loop and sub loop momentum for rejuvenation. Because of its unique dual purpose, capillary cell outer membranes and mitochondria flux permeability and combustion to stem and pace interstitial space sanitation, and rejuvenation of themselves and their interstitial space partners while facilitating an upgraded end organ function. The capillary cell outer membrane fluxing prevents chronic interstitial space inflammation thereby becoming a potent blocker of chronic illnesses, depleted end organ function and subsequent pain and fatigue.

Making energy utilizing electron transfer through the cytochromes is very efficient when compared to anaerobic methods. For each ATP molecule produced through cytochrome V, four hydrogen ions must emerge from the intermembrane space. Cytochrome V has the capacity to make up to one hundred ATP molecules per second, meaning it can process four hundred hydrogen molecules per second. One glucose molecule yields just four ATP molecules through anaerobic metabolism but at least 34 ATP (see appendix figure 6) through the mitochondrial matrix and cytochromes. Capillary cell mitochondria, along with their elaborate outer membrane receptor network, have allowed capillary cells to evolve an elaborate and potent immune surveillance system to serve the end organ and protect the interstitial space.

Capillary-Cell Outer Membranes

The most sophisticated, complex and elaborate set of outer-membrane receptors, pores and voltage gradients within any cell in the human body belongs to capillary cells. Capillary cell infrastructure comingles with three different outer membranes each containing different arrays of membrane infrastructure, receptors, pores and voltage gradients designed to protect the interstitial space and serve specific end organ function. Within these membranes are complex clumps of structural proteins, different densities and diversity of receptor proteins and pores, as well as variable levels of thickness, and voltage gradients. Together, they work in aggregate to texture and nuance permeability of blood plasma constituents to support interstitial space hygiene and end organ function. As previously discussed, capillary cell basement membrane anatomy can vary substantially from one end organ thereby conforming to specific end organ function. In contrast, capillary and endothelial cell outer membrane receptors on the luminal side of the cell have more uniformity as they must confer specific immune responses in mobilizing and immune response to inflammatory breach within the interstitial space regardless of where they reside.

Capillary cell outer membrane receptors must be both *dense and diverse* to implement a specific and sequenced immune arsenal response to an interstitial space inflammatory breach. When it comes to eliminating inflammation, the choreography of an immune arsenal response becomes critical. The detailing is facilitated by capillary cell outer membrane receptor specificity. Specificity enables recruitment and attachment of the right kind and volume of inflammatory mediator.

With so much at stake, persistent slipups in choreography detailing can be enough to provide advantage to chronic inflammation within the interstitial space. This can then trigger proinflammatory chain reactions that cascade disruption of interstitial space homeostasis, thereby opening the gate to the inflammatory matrix and a chronic inflammatory agenda.

Adjusting a sequenced permeability of immune arsenal into the interstitial space requires a specific reconfiguring of capillary cell outer membrane protein infrastructure. The reconfiguring, caused by the shifting and bending of infrastructure proteins, exposes different receptors enabling specific attachments of different remnants of immune arsenal arriving from the blood plasma. This nuances precision in the immune arsenal response to inflammatory breach to make it more likely that breach will be contained or eliminated. Thus exacting choreography becomes dependent on collected *accurate intelligence* about the inflammatory breach within the interstitial space, appropriate capillary cell outer membrane *receptor exposures*, an *optimal immune arsenal* arriving from blood plasma, and an ample *energy supply* to facilitate actively transport mechanics in the mobilization of the attached immune arsenal into the interstitial space.

Feedback Loops

Capillary cells—in fact, all cells—function in cascades of feedback loops, or chain reactions that build momentum to execute specific functions. This can be viewed as a series of turnkeys where one key unlocks another, which then unlocks another, and so on. Feedback loops can either stimulate or inhibit a function, often simultaneously, meaning they can turn on one while turning off another effect at the same time. This means a feedback loop or sub loop can act as both an *on and off switch*. The loop can turn one function on while simultaneously turning another function off. The basis for turning on and off switches simultaneously helps capillary cells and all cells regulate homeostasis and *balance* their different purposes. In this sense, being equally able to turn a given switch on and off helps the cell *redirect its purpose*. The more elegant the sub loops systems have evolved, the more nuanced the on-off switching becomes.

This can be viewed as akin to the difference between wakefulness and sleep. These are two very contrasting types of consciousness, but with optimal homeostasis of both, they each restore, integrate, and improve the functionality of the other. As a corollary, neither sleep nor wakefulness functions well without the other. So it is with feedback loops in capillary cells that facilitate an on-off switch system that supports adjustment in purpose, with each purpose supporting the other. In the big picture of capillary cell feedback loops, the capillary cell dance of permeability pivoting and combustion swinging connects immune surveillance and improved interstitial space hygiene to rejuvenation and augmented end organ function.

Feedback loops become dangerous when cascading imbalances create disparities in the on-off switch system. That is when switches are allowed to stay on or off for too long, they create momentum for adverse feedback loop damage. To use the example of the sleep wake cycle, if there is too much time spent in wakefulness and not enough time spent in sleep, derangements will occur in the quality of the wakefulness. Cognition, mental acuity and emotional disturbances will occur. For capillary cells, this feedback loop disruption will occur when there is excessive and persistent vascular free radical festering within the interstitial spaces. This persistently increases capillary cell outer membrane permeability, which feeds back a persistent "on" switch to mitochondrial energy combustion thereby creating cascades of adverse proinflammatory momentum within capillary cells. By blocking the ebb and flow of capillary and endothelial cell outer membrane permeability on-off switch feedback homeostasis is altered creating chain reactions of proinflammatory momentum within capillary cells, which extends to involve the interstitial space and the subsequent emergence of the inflammatory matrix and anti-organ.

When feedback loops build momentum to increase an effect, it is called *positive feedback,* whereas the off side of the switch is known as *negative feedback.* In the capillary cell, when momentum builds to a positive feedback, it simultaneously the same momentum to a negative feedback. When this persists, feedback loop imbalances occur that favor proinflammatory effects. A switch left on for too long means that another switch is left off. Flux is key to capillary cell sustenance, purpose and function. It implies that feedback loops but flux on and off as well.

In capillary-cell mitochondria, making efficient energy is important, but the *purpose* for making energy is more important. If the purpose supports successful *removal* of inflammatory momentum within interstitial spaces, capillary outer membrane fluxing and balanced feedback loop margins inspire optimal homeostasis. On the other hand, if capillary cell outer membranes have been hijacked as part of a conspiring takeover of the interstitial space by the inflammatory matrix, permeability flux is lost, positive and negative feedback loop relationships disrupted, and the capillary cell outer membranes become takeover targets to the highest bidder.

The mosaic of feedback-loop switches becomes constructive as to how capillary cells intuitively manage homeostasis that involves a multi- purpose. Optimal capillary-cell management of the end organ's interstitial space, rejuvenation of itself and its partners, as well as amplifying end-organ function requires a balanced and diametrically opposed set of feedback loop on –off switches that must flux in order to maintain optimal homeostasis. This enables the capillary cell to fulfill different purposes with cool and calculated efficiency.

Inflammatory Mediators

At any given time, the *capillary-cell outer-membrane complex*, is attracting and blocking different subsets of inflammatory mediators. They do this by reconfiguring their outer membranes receptors and pores while adjusting voltage gradients to accommodate different arrays of choreographed immune arsenal into the interstitial space. First-line or vascular inflammatory free radicals seed inflammation into the interstitial space, are driven by vulnerable genetics and potentiated by poor lifestyle choices. They include a variety of behaviors that limit exercise, impair sleep, induce stress, cause binge eating or drinking, or facilitate the use of cigarettes or drugs. Together and often in aggregate, they initiate and accelerate a diffuse multiple end organ interstitial space inflammation by penetrating into and through capillary-cell outer membranes to seed and attach to most anything within the interstitial space. As they fester, they induce chronic inflammation by employing the expansion of the immune arsenal which in this book is referred to as second line inflammatory mediators. They consist of white blood cells cytokines, complement, immunoglobulins and platelets. It is this group, along with mesenchymal cells, that chronic inflammation parlays propaganda to confuse their intent such that they become the problem rather than solution to the interstitial space.

Vascular inflammatory free radicals have been described elsewhere but include stress hormones, increases in shear membrane surface friction induced from hypertension, homocysteine, lipoprotein(a), oxidized LDL cholesterol, AGEs (from sugars), triglycerides, alcohol, and inhaled tobacco toxins (see appendix, graphs 1–5). The list of vascular inflammatory free radicals is growing. Its aggregate of vascular inflammatory free radical fall-out can often be determined by how much HSCRP (highly sensitive c reactive protein) is in the blood stream. The controlling influence to chronic inflammation and whether capillary cells can dance becomes dependent on the allotment of this group within interstitial spaces. Small amount of them in the interstitial space favor optimal capillary cell homeostasis, whereas larger volumes block there flux dance and disrupt homeostasis.

Like first line vascular inflammatory free radicals, second-line inflammatory mediators, *can work either for or against the capillary and end organ.* Smaller more precise movements of inflammatory mediators to contain and eliminate acute inflammatory breach work in favor of the capillary cell, end organ and interstitial space homeostasis. Larger volumes of persistent infusions of immune arsenal mobilized into the interstitial space create more risk for mistakes, breach of contract and confusion as to who they take instructions from. When they arrive from the blood plasma their intent is to contain and eliminate inflammatory breach. With chronic inflammation, once they get there messages get confused and intent blurs. With just a nudge and a bit of persuasion, they can switch allegiance.

To facilitate a sequenced immune arsenal response to an inflammatory breach, capillary cell outer membranes, with the help of energy supplied from mitochondria, reconfigure receptors to *attract, attach, bind, and roll* immune arsenal to *gap junctions, vesicles and transport channels* to create a specific response to eliminate the inflammatory breach. When chronic inflammation controls the interstitial space much of this choreography gets shelved and is replaced by a more random infusion of immune arsenal thereby perpetuating more chaos and the bait and switch in allegiance. This builds momentum to the takeover of capillary cell outer membranes utilizing the immune arsenal. Without really lifting a finger, the emerging inflammatory matrix builds on its momentum with preexisting parts.

The wheels fall off the capillary cell cart when sufficient numbers of mitochondria overheat and die (see appendix, figure 7), thereby losing large volumes within the cell. Without enough mitochondria or energy and no real stimulus for rejuvenation, the capillary cell shrivels including its outer membrane receptors, pore diversity and voltage gradients. This practically begs the interstitial space inflammatory matrix to pirate them. Fueled by vascular inflammatory free radicals, the inflammatory matrix seizes the capillary cell outer membranes without so much as a whimper in a bloodless coupe.

Just like the secret of chronic inflammatory expansion is to block the capillary cell dance, the secret to unblocking is to take away the fuel of chronic inflammation. Removing vascular free radicals starves chronic inflammation and takes the rust off of capillary cell outer membrane fluxing of their permeability. By doing so, they rejuvenate mitochondrial volumes, which become the backbone to resuscitating outer membrane receptor effectiveness. As arriving interstitial space immune arsenal regains focus to eliminate inflammatory breach, remnants of the matrix or anti-organ are either boxed in or go into hiding. This potentially enables capillary cell outer membranes to come all the way back an begin *fluxing permeability back and forth favoring their dance and optimize their homeostasis.* Reducing vascular inflammatory mediators (see appendix, graphs 1–5) becomes the hinge that could swing anti-inflammatory momentum enough to cause a renaissance of the capillary cell's intended purposes. Hello wellness.

The Glycolysis-Gluconeogenesis "Two-Step"

The capillary cell outer membrane permeability pivot -mitochondrial combustion pendulum swing dance is not the only two-step dance in the capillary cell. When probing energy requirements of capillary cells, most of what they need in carrying out usual cellular mechanics is generated within their cytoplasm by *glycolysis,* and countered by its sidekick partner, *gluconeogenesis.* Together they become important co -managers of pyruvate and glucose levels in capillary cells and to a large extent in all cells. Ninety percent of energy produced in capillary cells is from anaerobic (without oxygen) glycolysis and *not* from mitochondrial combustion. This allows capillary cell mitochondria the benefit of restricting energy combustion to surge requests from outer membranes to manage interstitial space sanitation. In this sense, glycolysis (where glucose is converted into pyruvate to yield 2 ATP molecules) can facilitate enough energy for the smooth management of running cytoplasm mechanics, facilitate glucose-pyruvate intracellular homeostasis, and supply pyruvate as fuel to mitochondria to cause production of acetyl CoA, which then can be utilized to combust energy or in the case of nitric oxide combustion, for protein synthesis.

When mitochondria are being bombarded with large amounts of fatty acids, pyruvate utilization is subverted. In this scenario which favors insulin resistance and diabetes, pyruvate is ushered back out of the mitochondria and is converted to glucose in the cytoplasm by gluconeogenesis.

The fact that capillary cells produce 90% of their total energy anaerobically speaks volumes in how they have adapted stingy oxygen utilization in order to nurture higher oxygen demands from end organs. Since end organs will always require more on demand oxygen to amplify their function, it only makes sense that capillary cells should not compete for the same arriving oxygen. Instead, capillary cell mitochondria utilize a fixed and small amount of oxygen, about 10% of what is delivered with the remainder diffusing into the interstitial space. Even in circumstances where nitric oxide increases blood flows to the capillary bed, they still will not use more than 10% of the total volume of oxygen delivered. Capillary cell glycolysis enables rationing of oxygen which then supports a more robust end organ function. This peculiarity to capillary cells has allowed end organs like the human brain to expand in size and capacity.

Both glycolysis and its inversion gluconeogenesis (see appendix, figure 8) involves a cumbersome ten-step process of fermentation. In glycolysis, glucose is metabolized to net two pyruvate and ATP molecules and two hydrogen ions, which attach to NAD (nicotinamide adenine dinucleotide) and are transported elsewhere or utilized if and when gluconeogenesis is required. Gluconeogenesis accomplishes the reverse when there are excessive volumes of pyruvate in the cell. Two pyruvate molecules come together to yield one glucose molecule, expending ATP in the conversion. This slow inefficient production of small volumes of energy that glycolysis provides, is in sharp contrast to the thirty plus ATP molecules that two pyruvate molecules produce in mitochondria when oxygen and the cytochrome system is utilized. Yet the genius is all of this is how well the capillary cell can function without the need for very much mitochondrial combustion utilizing oxygen.

Capillary-cell dependent glycolysis (and its antithesis, gluconeogenesis) provides important positive and negative feedback loops to mitochondrial combustion and ultimately to the end organ they serve. Their benefits include:

- Limiting capillary-cell oxygen combustion, thereby allowing more oxygen to diffuse to the oxygen-dependent end organs.
- (Glycolysis) glucose--pyruvate--glucose (gluconeogenesis) becomes an important regulator of pyruvate homeostasis in the cell's cytoplasm.
- By regulating capillary-cell cytoplasmic glucose-pyruvate metabolism, glycolysis and gluconeogenesis check-and-balance fatty-acid concentrations within the capillary cell as well.

By buffering pyruvate (and glucose) levels in the capillary cell glycolysis becomes an important cog in capillary-cell energy substrate homeostasis, while providing enough energy to capillary cells for the management of most operations that don't require outer membrane active transport or rejuvenation.

Mitochondrial Free Radicals: Friend, Foe, or Both?

Mitochondrial-exhaust here to fore known as reactive oxygen species (ROS) is defined as *free radicals* produced when mitochondria utilize oxygen to combust energy or nitric oxide. These free radicals can be toxic in the sense that some, such as when superoxide and hydrogen peroxide among others attach to membranes or DNA and do direct damage to them. At the same time, when ROS is produced as part of an energy surge to enable a sequenced uptick in immune arsenal mobilization into the interstitial space to eliminate an inflammatory breach, they can induce a beneficial adjustment to outer membrane permeability to further augment the inflammatory response.

On the other hand when produced in excess, and when participating in an uptick of non -sequenced immune arsenal response to chronic inflammation within the interstitial space, ROS attachments to membrane surfaces produce more harm than good. In this scenario, they enable an even more random immune arsenal exposure into the interstitial space thereby enabling the evolution of further chronic inflammatory organization. Hence just like with other feedback loops get unhinged, too much ROS from excessive mitochondrial energy combustion, and it will aid and abet the enemy.

Free radicals are ubiquitous, can form from a variety of different chemical reactions and as such can chain react to cause either pro or anti-inflammatory momentum. Proinflammatory momentum is more likely from free radical chain reactions when there is chronic interstitial space inflammation. In this scenario, the capillary dance is blocked, mitochondrial combustion stays in energy mode and superoxide free radical production intensifies. Not only do antioxidant levels diminish from overutilization, but superoxide related free radical chain reaction increase to double down on proinflammatory margins within the capillary cell. Thus the presence of increased superoxide increases damage by itself to endothelial and capillary cell membrane e and DNA surfaces as well as contributes to an increase in proinflammatory free radical chain reactions. All of these changes garner proinflammatory momentum that reduces capillary cell mitochondrial volumes and contributes to outer membrane pseudocapillarization. This becomes the ideal setup for the inflammatory matrix to pirate the capillary cell outer membranes utilizing the by now rogue interstitial space immune arsenal. Everything that was right side up, goes upside down when chronic inflammation changes the course of history in the interstitial space.

Superoxide free radicals by themselves are tough nuts to neutralize and require specific antioxidants housed and produced within the mitochondrial matrix. They also require a plethora of other more generic antioxidants to prevent secondary chain reactions that they can also induce. The antioxidants include families of *glutathione and manganese superoxide dismutase* (MnSOD), as well as the more generic antioxidants *vitamins E and C, alpha lipoic acid, coenzyme Q_{10}* (CoQ_{10}), and DHA/ EPA. The MnSOD group of antioxidants can reduce superoxide in combination with glutathione (glutathione peroxidase-GPX). The antioxidant combination reduces superoxide to hydrogen peroxide, which is then further reduced to carbon dioxide and water (see appendix, figure 10). Also in figure 10, superoxide exhaust can be seen to arise from energy combustion involving electron transfer from either the first or third cytochrome.

Superoxide exhaust does not occur from nitric oxide combustion. The exhaust from nitric oxide combustion can also be potentially toxic but not nearly as much as that of superoxide from energy combustion. In endothelial and capillary cells this is due to biased decreases in nitric oxide combustion that is directly linked to unmitigated interstitial space chronic inflammation.

All this discussion about ROS should make it clear that ROS can be a positive participant in the maintenance of the capillary cell dance and in optimal interstitial space homeostasis. It can also do catastrophic damage when overproduced from overheated mitochondrial energy combustion. Best results are always garnered when capillary cells are dancing and mitochondrial exhaust gets diversified from swinging back and forth. In this sense, pendulum swinging combustion creates a positive and negative antioxidant feedback loop that ensures toxic ROS can have a beneficial effect where it is supposed to but also gets neutralized before it does damage. By swinging mitochondrial combustion back and forth, ROS keeps its benefits while reducing its risks.

Figure 11 in the appendix summarizes the effects of chronic inflammation, persistent oxidative stress, and excessive superoxide

ROS production from too much mitochondrial energy combustion. In this depiction, escalating superoxide exhaust disrupts capillary-cell mechanics in a variety of ways to accelerate dysfunction. Figure 12 in the appendix depicts how chronic inflammation and increased oxidative stress (ROS production) can accelerate shortening of nuclear telomeres and increase DNA damage. The figure depicts a free-radical cross-linkage to nuclear chromosomes, which produces *gene silencing.* Gene silencing either reduces synthesis of or disrupts coding to such a degree that proteins are either not produced or have no function when they are. In the mitochondrial matrix, ROS can linger and damage naked mitochondrial DNA quickly, to produce draconian fission, abrupt suicide and rapid loss of volumes. Finally, ROS can even impact mRNA translation in ribosomes. This results in either a very defective or blocked protein synthesis. All of these effects become lethal to long term capillary cells health and favors the anti-organ strut within the interstitial spaces of end organs.

Chapter 4

THE TRIANGULAR INTERPLAY OF CAPILLARY-CELL MITOCHONDRIAL COMBUSTION, OUTER-MEMBRANE PERMEABILITY, AND THE IMMUNE ARSENAL

Up until the last thirty years, capillary cells were thought to be passive players in providing oxygen and nutrients to end organs. It was the end organ cell agenda that pushed cause and effect on the capillary cell and thus became the intuitive basis for disease treatment models involving end organ interventions. We now know that this is not even remotely true. We have come to understand that the interstitial space defines end organ health, that vascular free radicals fuel inflammation within that space, and that the immune arsenal that intervenes is controlled largely by capillary cell sequenced dispersal. This makes controlling chronic inflammation more important in wellness and prevention, as opposed to managing disease outcomes from end organs that in most instances have already been severely impacted by a well-organized anti-organ. I think even the casual observer can see that our current disease treatment model is late stage treatment and involves wrestling with complications from a long gone, out of the gate anti-organ venue(s). Wellness presupposes that interventions should occur before the anti-organ has advanced venues that have severely crippled the end organ-capillary cell relationship.

The capillary cell utilizes its dense outer-membrane receptor network and three different membrane surfaces to facilitate specific purposes of protecting the interstitial space and nurturing a specific end organ function. While their unique pore and basement-membrane development relative to specific end organ function may grab interest in disease treatment, when it comes to preventing chronic interstitial space inflammation it is the discovery of how capillary cells' mange the immune arsenal that emanates into the interstitial space that should garner the most intense interest. It is here that the battle for control of the interstitial space is lost or won. The capillary cell's capacity to maintain control of immune arsenal choreography, as it applies to the management of interstitial space hygiene defines anti-aging, predicts optimal end organ function and facilitates less fatigue and pain. Its capacity to do is best predicted by how well it is dancing which is directly attributable to the reduction of vascular inflammatory free radicals.

Let me summarize the factors that predict success or failure of capillary cell dancing.

- The *volume, diversity and persistence of* vascular inflammatory free radicals within the interstitial space.
- The *receptor capacity* of the capillary-cell outer membranes.
- The *volume* of capillary-cell mitochondria.
- The correct *pacing and, type of* immune arsenal dispersed to the inflammatory breach.
- The amount of chronic inflammatory *organization* that has occurred within the interstitial space. In other words is chronic inflammation in its early stages or has it organized enough to produce its own agenda (matrix) or venue(s) (anti-organ).

The last bullet forms the basis for the other four. When chronic inflammation establishes an interstitial space foothold, it organizes and forms agendas that disrupt immune dispersal, mitochondrial volumes and outer membrane receptors. It is fueled by vascular inflammatory free radicals. Eventually the predictable betrayal of the interstitial space immune arsenal and mesenchymal cells, coupled with pseudocapillarization of capillary cell outer membranes, sets up the capillary cell outer membrane hijacking by rogue immune arsenal. The gate then opens for anti-organ venues that cause serious diseases, compromise the end organ and cause debilitating pain and fatigue. It is at this late stage where disease treatment models intervene. It makes sense given the gravity of late inflammatory decline that has already occurred. Interventions at this stage are expensive, involve high tech, are wrought with complications, and usually require expensive surveillance and more interventions.

It can also be seen, that disease treatment is missing the boat. Finding treatment to remove amyloid, dissolve clots, remove thrombosis, resect cancers or treat infections while potentially lifesaving and well-intended, in the grand scheme, have not dealt with the elephant in the room-chronic inflammation fueled by vascular inflammatory free radicals. Ignoring the elephant set up recurring cycles of different anti-organ venues that can involve different end organs. A hip or knee can be replaced but progressive dementia from amyloid deposition and ischemic thrombosis preclude their benefits. Or a cardiac stent two or three are placed to stabilize angina and prevent a heart attack, only to have the blood thinners prescribed cause bladder bleeding, which then leads to a diagnosis of bladder cancer, surgery and chemotherapy. You get the point. Disease treatment does not prevent more interventions but rather nurtures them. In fact, many of us feel guilty if we have not had multiple interventions in any given year because we think something is wrong if we don't! Talk about twisted thinking. Even so, it is entirely predicted and even expected based on how disease treatment works.

Quality Assurance

The capacity of capillary-cell outer membranes to flux permeability and then swing mitochondrial combustion facilitates interstitial-space sanitation, while both refurbishing and optimizing end-organ function. Finding the sweet spot of the optimal capillary cell dual purpose is what defines effective *quality assurance*. It means that all feedback loops within the capillary cell, whether positive or negative, are working to effectively counterbalance on-off switches. Doing so actually makes the opposing loop function better. *Fluxing* defines optimal quality assurance and is best represented by the pivot and swing dance. All feedback loops and sub loops will follow suit.

It also implies that vascular inflammatory free radicals are tamed within interstitial spaces thereby permitting capillary cell outer membrane permeability pivoting. When tamed, the implication is that the feedback loop mosaic between capillary cells, downstream endothelial cells, the immune arsenal, mesenchymal and end organ cells is perfunctory.

Finally it means that the capillary cell dance ripples and paces positive anti-inflammatory momentum to protecting and optimizing the interstitial space, respond to end organ interests and to stem and pace rejuvenation to itself and its partners. Successful rejuvenation becomes the final exam to capillary cell quality assurance.

Quality assurance is breached by any persistent blockage of the capillary cell dance. In this sense, capillary cell quality assurance is dependent on its outer membrane flux, which is dependent on how much chronic inflammatory pestering is occurring within the interstitial space.

DNA Blueprints

In all cells with mitochondria, including capillary and endothelial cells, the *nucleus* and *mitochondria* within these cells both have coding *blueprints*. In contrast to nuclear DNA, the *mitochondrial DNA blueprint is naked*, meaning it lacks protection from a *telomere cap*. Naked DNA is inherently more vulnerable to free-radical cross-linkage. Since mitochondrial DNA is both naked and lies next to the combustion apparatus that produces free radical exhaust, it is in the direct line of fire to becoming disabled.

Mitochondrial DNA is particularly vulnerable to lingering superoxide free-radicals, which tend to accumulate with sustained energy combustion. When superoxide collides with mitochondrial DNA, it pushes cross linkage which degrades its capacity to code correctly.

Over time the accumulation of cross linkage induces mitochondrial fission, suicide and loss of volumes within the capillary cell. The loss of mitochondria within endothelial and capillary cells provides proinflammatory momentum towards pseudocapillarization of its outer membranes and a more random colonization of the interstitial space of unwanted immune arsenal. This eventually leads to the so called capillary cell zombie state and enables the chronic inflammatory matrix to pirate the outer membrane complex.

Mitochondrial DNA contains the blueprints for coding proteins for only some of its infrastructure and inner membrane cytochromes. Therefore, code quality and its effect on mitochondrial protein replacements are shared with nuclear DNA. If coding is poor or erratic due to superoxide or free radical damage (oxidative stress), the replacement proteins are either not replaced or function comparatively worse than those they are intended to replace. In mitochondria, this leads to fission and suicide.

The risk for damaged DNA, nuclear or mitochondrial, becomes dependent on getting rid of mitochondrial exhaust quickly. This requires abundant antioxidants and limited accumulation of one type or kind of free radical. The best way of accomplishing both is through fluxing of outer membrane permeability and swinging mitochondrial combustion back and forth. This diversifies free radical exhaust and enables antioxidants to re accumulate and not be over utilized.

The mitochondrial remedies (see appendix, figure 7) to DNA cross linkage are draconian as diminished mitochondrial capacity just fuels capillary cell declines. The only spark towards reversal requires and injection of lifestyle turnabout.

Keeping naked mitochondrial DNA from degrading by fluxing capillary cell outer membrane permeability requires suitable lifestyle choices that permeate wellness.

Homeostasis

Endothelial and capillary-cell homeostasis is a moving target and by its nature is subject to risk due to how much integration of information the complex outer membrane receptor network must facilitate. That facilitation coupled with constant adjustments in interstitial space hygiene and oxygen-nutrient demands from end organ create real time shifts to feedback loops and on-off switches. In this setting, *homeostasis* refers to how well a cell can center itself given its how it must adjust moment to moment. How facile a capillary cell can adjust truly depends on the mechanics of its feedback loops, which at its core, requires the flux dance between its outer membranes and mitochondria.

Fluxing to maintain homeostasis becomes *counterintuitive*, as homeostasis becomes dependent on how well sanitation of the interstitial space is managed. Sanitation becomes dependent on vascular free radical volumes, there persistence and how much they have enabled organization of chronic inflammation. If interstitial space sanitation is maintained at a high level, capillary cell outer membranes will flux permeability, mitochondrial will swing combustion and all the feedback loop on- off switches that follow will properly coordinate optimal homeostasis.

Optimal endothelial and capillary cell homeostasis also implies not just an intimacy with its interstitial space and end organ cells, but also an *intuitive interconnectedness* between all other cells outside of their interstitial space orbit, including other capillary and downstream endothelial cells as well as other end-organ cells.

Optimal capillary cell homeostasis is shifted when any of the moving components mentioned above is impairing outer membrane flux. Without reduction in proinflammatory mediators, the tug of war for control of capillary cell outer membranes will not be favorable to capillary cell homeostasis. When capillary cell homeostasis flounders, proinflammatory momentum prevails, chronic illnesses escalate, end organs decline and waves of fatigue and debilitating pain punctuate the clinical landscape.

Calcium Ions

In the capillary cell, *calcium ion flux* in and out of mitochondria, as a result of combustion pendulum swinging, is a key modulator in the execution of outer-membrane permeability adjustments. In capillary cells stored calcium ions, within mitochondria and adjacent smooth endoplasmic reticulum, are released in conjunction with mitochondrial energy combustion. Calcium along with ATP, migrate to capillary cell out membranes to stump an increase in permeability of immune arsenal through capillary-cell outer membranes to and from the interstitial spaces of end organs. Calcium ions work through pumps and different enzymes that act as on –off switches on capillary cell outer membranes to enable permeability adjustments. Calcium adjusts permeability by decreasing outer membrane voltage gradients, facilitating actin-myosin fibril sliding to reshape the capillary cell outer membrane to oval, and my facilitating adjustments in outer membrane infrastructure thereby exposing different sets of receptor surfaces for immune arsenal attachment. All of these outer membrane adjustments facilitate movement of inflammatory mediators into the interstitial space.

When done properly, meaning without chronic inflammatory influence, the release of calcium ions by mitochondria allows capillary-cell outer membrane's to set the table for a sequenced immune arsenal response to remove an interstitial space inflammatory breach. As calcium ions leave the mitochondrial matrix, they uncouple from phosphate, making more phosphorus available in the conversion of ADP to ATP. The newly minted negatively charged ATP is then coupled with positively charged magnesium and transported out of the mitochondrial matrix to be deposited at capillary cell outer membranes to facilitate active transport of inflammatory mediators through channels, vesicles or the gap junction into the interstitial space.

When inflammatory breach is eliminated—and the salient word here is *eliminated*—calcium is no longer required to increase outer-membrane permeability for additional inflammatory mediators to enter the interstitial space. With the down ward shift in capillary cell outer membrane permeability, calcium ions transition back to the mitochondrial matrix, setting up a reversal in outer membrane voltage gradients, actin- myosin fibril sliding and membrane protein bending. As calcium ions build within the cytoplasm and then reenter into the mitochondria, they help facilitate activation of nitric oxide synthetase. This activation shuts down electron transfer through the cytochrome system thereby effectively blocking mitochondrial energy combustion. As capillary cell combustion converts to nitric oxide, calcium ions once again build up and are stored in the mitochondrial matrix and adjacent smooth endoplasmic reticulum. Capillary cell outer-membranes convert from oval to flat to accommodate greater exposures to the end organ. As capillary cells flatten out, their gap junction orifices and channels narrow and their vesicles and transport channels become less active.

As calcium ions move back into the mitochondrial matrix they are exchanged through the inner membrane with combinations of hydrogen, sodium, and magnesium which facilitates inner membrane voltage mechanics.

To summarize, calcium ion storage (linked to nitric oxide combustion) and release (linked to energy combustion) in the capillary-cell mitochondrial matrix is a powerful feedback loop modifier tied to:

- The pendulum swinging of mitochondrial combustion.
- Outer membrane actin-myosin fibril sliding (contraction).
- Adjustments in gap junction orifice and channel width.
- Exposure to end organ cell outer membranes
- Capillary cell outer-membrane and mitochondrial inner membrane voltage gradients.
- The execution of the capillary cell dance.

Inflammatory Mediators: How They Destroy What They Are Supposed to Preserve

Capillary-cell mitochondria and outer membranes interlock with feedback loops to protect the interstitial space, facilitate a specific end organ function, and stem/ pace rejuvenation for itself and its interstitial space partners. As long as capillary cells can flux outer membrane permeability without undue constraints, these processes are seamless and allow for the expansion or contraction of inflammatory responses within interstitial spaces as well as the nurturing and rejuvenation of the end organ. The *reach* of capillary cell outer membrane fluxing of permeability can include a broad array of different inflammatory expanders. In addition to white blood cells, complement, platelets, immunoglobulins and cytokines, can also include various families of *growth factors. The primary purpose of growth factors is to address end organ duress. This usually involves inadequate oxygen supplies and is addressed by attempts to increase blood flow to the end organ.* Unfortunately, growth factors can also be sued by the anti-organ in chronic inflammation to drive cancer growth.

The fact is any of the immune arsenal can be used by the anti-organ for its venues, but growth factors (for example, vasoactive endothelial growth factor-VEGF) are a prime example of how immune arsenal can act on behalf of the end organ or conversely for the anti-organ. Growth factors do different things based on where they come from and when they are released. In capillary cells growth factors can increase capillary-cell mitosis to cause growth of new blood vessels (angiogenesis) to theoretically increase blood flow (and oxygen) to the end organ. Capillary angiogenesis can work if downstream vessels can dilate their lumens to increase blood flow through them. If they can't increase their lumens due to too much stiffness (basement membrane thickening) or obstructive plaque, capillary cell angiogenesis upstream does not work, unless they can finagle more blood flow from *collateral circulation*. In this case, capillary cells support angiogenesis by *importing* or diverting blood from other large downstream blood vessels. This could backfire as the imported blood may have been needed where it was intended to go originally, but nonetheless diverting blood flow gives capillary cells a chance to succeed with angiogenesis. It will also not work if capillary and other cells have been zombie by the anti-organ and growth factors are being produced and utilized to expand anti-organ intent, such as with cancer growth.

With chronic inflammation within interstitial spaces, growth factors can also be used by the anti –organ directly or indirectly to increase their venues. The classic example is for cancer growth, but they can also use growth factors to support autoimmune complex disease and the seeding of bacterial infections.

Persistent exposures within the interstitial space of any combination of vascular inflammatory free radicals, fuel chronic inflammation, enable the inflammatory matrix and create opportunity for white blood cells, cytokines, immunoglobulins, complement and platelets within the interstitial space to switch allegiance. The double agent effect makes immune arsenal a potential deadly advocate for the emerging anti-organ. Thing get very bad in a hurry when immune arsenal begins working for the enemy.

At first blush the immune arsenal gyration in loyalty would appear as an unexpected coupe. In retrospect the betrayal should have been intuitively obvious. The fact is, the capillary cell had been rendered irrelevant and essentially incompetent in managing its own affairs. With just a basic shell of mitochondria and outer membrane receptors it had becomes nothing more than a vacant ship at sea waiting to be seized. At this stage, it would only make sense that the proinflammatory momentum provided by the chronic inflammatory matrix would prove too enticing for either the immune arsenal or mesenchymal cells to ignore. Now instead of taking out inflammatory breach, they promote facilitating chronic inflammatory milieus within the interstitial space that foster scarring, cancer, infections, autoimmune disorders and thrombosis. All of this unhinges the end organ, and increases pain, fatigue and aging.

In this manner, the capillary cell becomes tortured by its previous allies. Whichever is the terminal event of choice employed by the anti-organ as a kill shot to the end organ, the die is being cast and is facilitated by the immune arsenal.

Chapter 5

HOW THE CAPILLARY-CELL DANCE OF "PIVOTING AND SWINGING" MAKES THE END ORGAN "SWING AND PIVOT"

Overview

Something should be clear by now: end organs are not the swashbuckling provocateurs that control their own destiny as was once thought. While they do make their demands known with a loud and resounding voice, what they actually get is dependent on how well capillary cells are dancing.

For the capillary cell to facilitate the end organ it must be able to adroitly multi task purpose. Its dense outer-membrane receptor-voltage gradient-pore system must be fully operational and its mitochondria completely revitalized. It's glycocalyx should be thick and basement membrane free or free radical debris. This requires minimizing free radical influences within the interstitial space and a rigorous capillary cell outer membrane fluxing of permeability and swinging of mitochondrial combustion. It is this penultimate feedback loop that supports all others both within and without the capillary cell. The pivot and swing co-depend on each other's function to make each other's function better. It becomes the secret to rejuvenation which keys remissions from chronic illness, reduces fatigue and pain, while becoming the true anti-aging tonic.

Besides outer membrane flux, capillary cells utilize other tricks in the maintenance of interstitial space sanitation. By keeping the their glycocalyx, thick and voltage gradients elevated, by sustaining pore and receptor density, and by ensuring competent vesicle and channel transport systems, outer membrane can sequence effective immune surveillance of the interstitial space. When healthy, capillary-cell outer membranes *prioritize hygiene* of the interstitial space, which ensures a more capable response to end organ demands.

Minimizing inflammatory-mediator free-radical exposures becomes the quintessential way of providing insurance that capillary cell's will be able to provide effective interstitial space hygiene. When capillary cells dance, the implication is that all endothelial and capillary cells throughout the arterial tree are capable of dancing. What is also true is the reverse. An identifiable blocked dance involving one end organ probably means similar patterns elsewhere and subsequent compromises to their interstitial spaces. Thus all end organ function is either augmented or suppressed when the endothelia of the entire vascular tree is dancing or not dancing. This makes what we eat, smoke and how we move and sleep as important as anything to break the potential stranglehold of chronic inflammation, as it correlates directly with how well endothelia are dancing.

When capillary cells dance, their powerful feedback loops pace dancing to mesenchymal and end organ cells. When capillary cells don't dance, *neither do mesenchymal or end organ cells but the anti-organ does.* When it comes to the capillary end organ relationship, capillary outer membrane permeability fluxing and mitochondrial pendulum swinging go in opposite directions. When capillary cell outer membranes s flux permeability downward, end organ cells flux their outer membrane permeability in the opposite direction to increase function. As this occurs, capillary mitochondria swing combustion to nitric oxide to rejuvenate while also providing impetus for nitric oxide driven increases in blood flow to the end organ.

The ability to shift purpose from interstitial space sanitation to augmenting end organ function and visa- versa means that capillary cells answer to both mesenchymal and end organ cells equally. This delicate and unique homeostasis has evolved on the basis of how capillary cells dance. When end organs increase combustion, they make waste products, which eventually accumulate to create a sanitation issue within the interstitial space. This requires capillary cells to pivot permeability and swing combustion to energy enable cleanup. As they do this, the end organ has quieted combustion of energy, reduced their outer membrane permeability and has swung combustion to nitric oxide to facilitate rejuvenation. All of this is paced and supported by the capillary endothelium. The pivot and swing from the capillary cell paces the end organ swing and pivot.

The Battle for Capillary-Cell Permeability Ownership

The presence or absence of the capillary cell pivot and swing determines the presence or absence of end organ swing and pivot. Its presence makes the end organ function better. Its absence pushes chronic inflammatory agendas, increases chronic illnesses, reduces end organ function and produces waves of fatigue and pain. In the case of the capillary cell, the pacing of the pivot and swing to the end organ's swing and pivot depends on who owns capillary cell outer membrane permeability. Ownership becomes a tug-of-war between the forces of good and evil within the interstitial space. If chronic inflammation wins, the stage is set for a pivot and swing capillary cell vacuum. If they don't, the pivot and swing reverberates through the entire interstitial space and beyond. When the deed of capillary cell outer membrane permeability ownership is transferred to the inflammatory matrix, it in effect surrenders control of the interstitial space, immune arsenal and mesenchymal cells. The space becomes the darling to the whims and venues of the emerging anti-organ, at the expense of the true end organ.

The hijacking of capillary cell outer membrane receptors by white blood cells and cytokines that have switched allegiance becomes the coup de –tat to the capillary cell and end organ. The immune arsenal moving into the interstitial space now have little or nothing to do with sanitation and more to do with propping up anti-organ venues.

Outer-Membrane Pores, Diaphragms and the Like

With few exceptions, capillary cells have a variety of different-sized outer-membrane pores and diaphragms to accommodate movement of a diverse molecular constituency into a given end organ's interstitial space. As inflammation within interstitial spaces becomes chronic, pores and diaphragms lose diversity to appear more as a generic "one size fits all". This generic momentum fits with other "adaptations" the capillary cell applies as mitochondrial volumes diminish and energy supplies for active transport dry up. These include reductions in outer membrane voltage gradients and receptor diversity, as well as glycocalyx thinning as basement membranes thicken. The sum aggregate of these changes dampens capillary outer membrane responsiveness to sequence immune arsenal properly into the interstitial space. What is not sequenced is allowed to enter the interstitial space randomly. This bodes poorly for the future of the interstitial space.

When capillary cell outer membrane permeability does not flux, outer-membranes eventually drop all the apparatus that makes them unique. When pores and diaphragms become one size or thickness, the flexibility of ushering specific proteins or filtering selectively through different diaphragms different mixes of electrolytes or other small molecules to nuance permeability is lost. *Uniform pores and diaphragms* on capillary cell membrane surfaces sharply limits a detailed immune arsenal entry into the interstitial space favoring an unfocused response to breach and enabling additional chronic inflammation.

Outer-Membrane Receptor Network

The basis for optimal capillary-cell outer membrane function is primarily the result of how it has evolved a massive and diverse group of receptors that become exposed to yield specific immune arsenal responses to inflammatory interstitial space beach. Receptors work best when used but not abused. This means that there are periods where they can be repaired or replaced. This is best performed when the pivot and swing dance enables nitric oxide combustion.

Capillary-cell outer-membrane receptors are a diverse group, interacting with its end organ, other end organs, interstitial-space mesenchymal cells, inflammatory mediators, adjacent capillary cells, as well as other endothelial cells of the arterial, venous, and lymphatic trees. Membrane receptors also respond to inbound and outbound immune arsenal, electrolyte shifts, albumin concentrations, fluctuating energy substrates as well as to changes in hydrostatic and osmotic pressures.

Capillary and endothelial cell receptors are composed of families of different enzymes and proteins that send and receive signals, attach cells and proteins from the blood plasma, and act as on/off switches, all of which increase or decrease outer membrane permeability. They often become exposed on capillary cell membrane surfaces through changes in structural membrane protein reconfiguration. Receptors become available based on interstitial space signals. Capillary cell luminal outer membrane surfaces can then attach different white blood cells, platelets, cytokines, and proteins based on the signal. Permeability is further nuanced by membrane on-off switches and voltage gradients, and the relative opening or closing of gap junction orifices and other transport channels. Executing the will of capillary-cell outer-membrane receptors requires a kindred relationship with adjacent mitochondria to supply calcium and energy for execution of nuanced outer membrane function.

To be effective in stratifying an inflammatory response to the interstitial space, outer membrane receptor density and diversity must be maintained. This will not occur without outer membrane permeability fluxing that is typical of chronic interstitial space inflammatory breach. Fluxing permeability permits increases the likelihood of proper repair and maintenance of membrane receptors.

Energy Driven Transcellular Transport

When interstitial spaces scream for the rapid movement of inflammatory mediators or albumen they harness the capillary cell receptor network to supply what they need. The transport of what they need is often accomplished by surges of energy from adjacent mitochondria. Energy drives outer membrane active-transport systems involving *vesicle endocytosis* and *trans- capillary transport channels*. In addition, capillary-cell outer membranes adjust pores, diaphragms, gap-junction orifices, receptor configurations, and the thickness of their glycocalyx and basement membranes in deference to a rapid energy driven mobilization of immune arsenal and proteins into the interstitial space. Utilizing an optimal energy surge, for specific immune arsenal transcellular transport from blood plasma to the interstitial space, can only be supplied by adjacent mitochondria.

The "channeling" of specific inflammatory mediators by energy-driven active-transport processes to facilitate elimination of inflammatory interstitial space breach actually becomes a potent feedback loop to generate an eventual downshift in capillary cell outer membrane permeability. The lack of a mitochondrial energy surge, when called upon, predisposes to the opposite. Most important the better the energy surge in supplying active transport of essential immune arsenal for removal of inflammatory breach, the more likely the subsequent nitric oxide response will be in supporting repair, maintenance of capillary cell infrastructure, mitochondrial volumes and outer membrane receptors. Energy supports interstitial space sanitation which supports rejuvenation which then supports interstitial space sanitation.

Outer-Membrane Voltage Gradients and Pumps

All capillary-cell outer membranes (including the *glycocalyx, continuous outer membrane,* and *basement membrane*) maintain some level of barrier support between blood plasma, capillary-cell cytoplasm, and the end-organ interstitial space. In part, the capillary cell barrier is created by how thick the glycocalyx or basement membrane is at a given moment coupled with the presence or absence of membrane slits or gaps, the tightness of their gap junctions, and how much voltage gradient the membrane employs. All of these membrane elements support a balance between what does and does not enter the interstitial space given the specific function of the end organ and the sanitation of the interstitial space.

Capillary cell outer membranes block molecular movement from blood plasma in part by creating electric currents across their membrane surfaces. The higher the current, the more *resistance* there is to crossing the membrane and the less permeability there is for molecular constituents to move through it. Higher voltage gradients are often a reflection in the activity of the outer membrane's potassium and sodium *pumps*. When calcium ions flood these pumps the potassium-sodium pump is blocked and membrane permeability increases as the voltage gradient decreases. Therefore, the flooding of calcium ions onto membrane surfaces plays an important role of increasing the capability of different types of immune arsenal movement into or out of the interstitial space. Calcium ions cascade numerous feedback loops at the outer membrane level, including the activation of actin-myosin fibril sliding and on -off switches to increase membrane permeability to inflammatory mediators.

Capillary cell outer voltage gradients are dependent on swinging mitochondrial combustion and at the same time mitochondrial combustion is dependent on voltage gradients to shift permeability to enable the swing in the opposite direction. Both are dependent on vascular inflammatory free radicals in the interstitial space and the presence of chronic inflammation.

Baseline outer membrane voltage gradients, as well as the absolute flux of electric currents through them, decrease with capillary cell pseudocapillarization. The reduced voltage gradients are not compensated for by other feedback loop adjustments. This results in an expected more random display of inflammatory mediators entering the interstitial space to cascade more immune miscues and expand chronic inflammation.

Actin-Myosin Fibrils

Attached strategically to the capillary-cell continuous outer membrane are small fibrils of actin and myosin. In the presence of calcium ions and energy, these fibrils are activated and slide on each other, causing a contraction. As fibrils contract in unison, they change the configuration of the capillary cell from flat to oval, thereby *opening up the gap-junction orifices* and *channels* on either side of the capillary cell to inflammatory-mediator movement from blood plasma to the interstitial space. The sliding of actin-myosin fibrils represents another mechanism that capillary cells utilize to increase outer membrane permeability to inflammatory mediators entering the interstitial space.

In order to slide optimally, they must receive energy and calcium from mitochondria. With less energy and calcium availability as might be seen with reduced mitochondrial volumes, actin myosin sliding becomes less robust fixating the capillary cell's outer membrane morphology into a generic looking partially flat morphology. This neither supports interstitial space hygiene or end organ function. If anything, the "tweener" morphology dampens capillary cell intent and pushes inflammatory momentum towards a more generic mistake prone immune arsenal entering the interstitial space. The inability to become completely oval and subsequently revert to completely flat is one more dagger to capillary cell integrity.

Nuclear Telomeres

In capillary cells, DNA is found in two locations, its nucleus and mitochondria. In contrast to nuclear DNA, mitochondrial chromosomal DNA lacks the protective *telomere cap, making it more vulnerable to free radical damage compared to nuclear DNA.* As such, with chronic inflammation within interstitial spaces, it is the non -capped mitochondrial DNA that is most at risk.

In the nucleus, the chromosomal DNA can still get damaged and often does so with aging and exposure to free radicals over time. Nuclear DNA contains a protective telomere cap, whose length and hence level of protection to chromosomes, is maintained by the enzyme *telomerase*. Telomerase can regenerate the telomere cap when capillary cells are stimulated to rejuvenate through mitochondrial nitric oxide combustion. On the other hand, telomere shortening accelerates with chronic interstitial space inflammation as capillary mitochondria spend less time in nitric oxide combustion. When they do combust nitric oxide, there are fewer of them making nitric oxide thereby limiting their effectiveness in activating telomerase activity.

As DNA s damage moves forward, when protein synthesis does occur, more coding mistakes are made and miss fitted proteins with little or no function result. This leads to further "silencing of intent" to capillary cell outer membrane receptors and other membrane surfaces involving mitochondria and other organelles when proteins are replaced. This means that replacement proteins, regardless of where they reside, can't or don't respond due to being malformed. In the case of capillary cell outer membranes, receptor silencing breeds more pseudocapillarization, creating a relapsing progression to chronic interstitial space inflammation. Increasingly defective capillary cell mitochondrial and nuclear DNA becomes a trap as well as a mechanism of anti-organ enablement.

The best way for telomerase to increase regeneration of nuclear telomeres is to nurture the capillary cell dance. A robust capillary cell dance helps to shift mitochondrial combustion to nitric oxide on a more regular basis thereby enabling not only telomerase activation but also more time being activated. This gives telomere lengthening and DNA protection half a chance. The same holds true for end organ cell telomeres as they dance in the opposite direction.

By kicking interstitial space inflammatory momentum to the curb, capillary cell outer membranes are afforded the opportunity to flux permeability triggering mitochondrial nitric oxide combustion which then sparks activation of telomerase. Lengthening telomeres does not solve the pre- existing DNA cross linkage problem, but it could prevent or at least slow DNA damage progression. Perhaps anti-inflammatory behaviors could actually stem nuclear DNA healing. If not, at least stabilizing nuclear DNA, by lengthening their telomeres, could make the difference in how proteins are coded, which eventually impacts the effectiveness of the pivot and swing and swing and pivot.

The Reach to End-Organ Quality Assurance and Homeostasis through Paced Capillary Cell Outer Membrane- Mitochondrial Dancing

Built-in quality performance by all end organs becomes dependent on contented capillary cells. Capillary cell contentment becomes dependent on interstitial-space hygiene. Limiting interstitial space free-radical inflammatory fall-out from excessive stress hormones, polluted air and tobacco toxins, alcohol, drugs, LDL cholesterol and AGEs among others, reduces proinflammatory momentum within the interstitial space creating opportunity for a revival of capillary cell pivoting and swinging. Enabling a steady diet of virulent vascular free radicals entering the interstitial spaces, pushes chronic inflammatory momentum and blocks the capillary cell pivot and swing dance.

Resetting the capillary cell dance has its earliest effects on improving mitochondrial volumes and replenishing outer membrane receptors, which then begins the process of revamping the influx of immune arsenal into the interstitial space. These initial improvements within capillary cells enable some interstitial space cleanup of chronic inflammatory residues. This is accomplished by gradually reassembling all the pieces to the capillary cell armamentarium within the interstitial space that had fallen astray as a result of chronic inflammatory influences. As interstitial space hygiene improves, increasingly, immune arsenal and mesenchymal cells become friendly with capillary cells once again. With additional anti-inflammatory momentum the residuals of the anti-organ go into isolation or solitary confinement as many of its malignant venues of chronic illnesses go into remission.

As the interstitial space heals, the capillary cell then rediscovers intimacy with its end organ partner. As they reconnect their feedback loop relationships are rediscovered, meaning the capillary cell pivot and swing becomes once again linked to the swing and pivot of the end organ.

As capillary cells dance, their dancing paces it partners within its orbit not only dance but dance better. The darkness of the interstitial space is replaced by rejuvenation. Most important, cataclysmic end-organ illnesses are shelved and pain, fatigue and aging become an asterisk. The fountain of youth becomes a dance from a most unsuspecting partner.

Chapter 6

INTERSTITIAL-SPACE WHITE FLAGS

Interstitial-space white flags represent the end game venues of the anti-organ. They amount to a surrender of the interstitial space to the dark forces, with their progression or recurrence forcing either severe compromise or death to the end organ. White flags occur when the anti-organ gains full control of the interstitial space and can use all known assets within the space to perpetuate its destructive purpose. It does this by exploiting the successful agenda of the chronic inflammatory matrix that came before it. The inflammatory matrix essentially created a capillary cell death triangle of reduced mitochondrial volumes, *pseudocapillarization* of their outer membranes, and increased cross-linkage of its DNA by blocking the capillary cell dance. In the process, it converted interstitial space immune arsenal and mesenchymal cells to its purpose. This enabled a hostile takeover of the capillary cell outer membranes by the newly converted immune arsenal. With the combination of the capillary cell death triangle and the pirating of their outer membranes, the inflammatory matrix passes the baton to the anti-organ to implement venues within the interstitial space that doom the end organ to a similar fate as the capillary cell.

All of this progression to the anti-organ starts innocently with the sprinkling of vascular inflammatory free radicals within interstitial spaces. Unfortunately, the initial sprinkling can become insidious and progressive often leading to a hoard. Given enough time, penetration and addiction, the initial sprinkling becomes a chronic inflammatory process within the interstitial space. With progression, chronic inflammatory influences coalesce and begin to mess with the capillary cell dance. With enough of a dance block, the process of mitochondrial meltdown begins and proinfalmmatory chain reactions to the capillary cell's outer membranes, organelles and DNA intervene.

As an example of vascular inflammatory innocence, let's look at a cigarette. This same argument that I am about to make can also be made for a donut, alcohol, narcotics, amphetamines or any addictive substance. As a teen smoking a cigarette would appear to a right- of passage. But there is one problem. Tobacco has nicotine and nicotine is very addictive. Even after just one cigarette, there is a desire to smoke more. Before you can blink twice, it escalates to a pack a day. Smoking just one cigarette does introduce 16 different inhaled proinflammatory substances into the bloodstream, which can penetrate interstitial spaces in multiple end organs. These can be cleared in their entirety by a capillary cell sequenced immune response without too much ado. Smoking a pack a day over a period of time is just too much free radical interstitial space penetration for the capillary cell to resolve. Chronic inflammation finds a beach head.

What is worse is that the proinflammatory effects escalate with age. Smoking one pack of cigarettes a day at age 60 is like smoking 3 packs at age 25. This is because of the persistent magnitude of toxicity that tobacco smoke causes in the bloodstream in a 60 year old. In other words, the smoke free radicals, increase in the interstitial space to a greater magnitude and with less resistance to them, enabling them to cause more direct membrane damage and accelerate anti-organ venues to the end organ.

Addiction to toxic substances is an example of how interstitial spaces can be invaded to chronically inflame the space, block the capillary cell dance and create an inflammatory matrix agenda. In the case of chronically inhaled cigarette smoke, most would connect the dots to the cause and effect of smoking to breathlessness, cough, lung cancer, emphysema and even heart conditions. But what they may not connect is the increased risk for dementia, disabling arthritis pain, amputation of a limb, rupture of an aneurysm, osteoporosis, disseminated infections, pneumonia, as well as cancers of the breast, prostate, colon, esophagus, stomach and pancreas. Smoking may also increase risk for autoimmune diseases and gastrointestinal bleeding from ulcers. The fact is, smoking causes a blocked capillary cell dance everywhere in the body which leads to different but malignant anti-organ venues in these different places. Addictions don't compartmentalize or isolate to a single end organ. Inflammation is occurring everywhere and every end organ is at risk for an anti-organ venue.

Adult diabetes, or even prediabetes, produces many of the same kinds of end organ complications over time that smoking does. Instead of inhaling 16 different toxins, adult diabetes produces a vast metabolic array of proinflammatory free radicals, each of which can assault membrane surfaces in any interstitial space, expand an immune arsenal inflammatory response towards them, and eventually enable chronic inflammation to form a matrix and block the capillary cell dance. Not only do elevated blood sugars disrupt intracellular glycolysis-gluconeogenesis homeostasis to favor gluconeogenesis, but they also increase free radicals such as AGEs, oxidized LDL cholesterol, triglycerides, and other low density non HDL cholesterols, as well as other circulating proinflammatory proteins. As basement membranes of endothelial cells thicken and become stiff, shear through their lumens increases and hypertension becomes an early and predictable outcome from diabetes. When diabetes, hypertension and high LDL cholesterol are co-linked, the interstitial space becomes an overt white flag of thrombotic risk.

This chapter will discuss anti-organ venues within the interstitial space that eventually become the death rattle to end organs. These venues are not unexpected and form the basis for most disease treatment models in the way medicine has been practiced over the past two hundred years. Unfortunately they also represent late outcomes to chronic inflammation and could largely be prevented if wellness and prevention nipped chronic inflammation earlier in the bud. When the anti-organ unleashes its venues, the end organ is always compromised which means there will be waves of fatigue and pain. A common venue to chronic inflammation is scarring, which can become a gateway to other anti-organ venues.

Fibrous Scar Tissue

In normal wound healing, the production of scar tissue is temporary and adaptive, as it forms a protective cap and seal while *normal tissue* grows back into the injured space. The scar tissue then sloughs when it is no longer required, leaving behind a repaired and fully functioning end-organ tissue. This can be observed from a skin cut or abrasion. The skin heals from the dermis inside to the epidermis outside, to eventually slough the scab cap thereby exposing new skin. This type of temporary scar formation is beneficial because the end organ is repaired and remains functional where the repair occurred.

However in chronic inflammation, the formation of fibrous scar tissue has a much different outcome. In this case, the scar does not slough to be replaced by normal end organ tissue, but instead *permanently replaces* normal end-organ tissue. This replacement becomes a predictable event when chronic inflammation within the interstitial space festers over an extended period of time, up to 20 or more years. Examples include cirrhosis scarring of the liver from chronic alcohol exposure, emphysema or COPD of the lung from chronic tobacco exposure, and amyloid scarring of the brain associated with dementia (Alzheimer's disease) from chronic diabetes and LDL cholesterol exposures. In all these examples, scarring is a late anti-organ venue that occurs from chronic exposures of vascular inflammatory free radicals.

Each end organ is vulnerable to different sets of white flag venues. For example, in the heart and brain, scar tissue comes becomes a predictable event based on inadequate supplies of oxygen delivery due to downstream larger vessel basement membrane thickening, obstructive plaque or thrombosis, all of which play out from persistent free radical seeding of the interstitial spaces over a period of time. It really does not matter if the seeding involves toxins from smoke or alcohol or from diabetes or LDL cholesterol.

What does matter is persistence. As heart and brain cells atrophy or die off, they are replaced by scar tissue as the end organ deteriorates its function. In the liver sinusoid or kidney glomerulus, scar tissue can accumulate as a result of chronic diabetes or LDL inflammation (fatty liver to cirrhosis and glomerular basement membrane sclerosis) but can also occur from repeated toxin exposures. Examples include chronic alcohol exposures to the liver and chronic acetaminophen exposure to the liver or the kidney glomerulus. The point is that many different types of chronic inflammation within end organ interstitial spaces can induce end organ scarring. And the anti-organ can employ different venues to cause other added on venues. For example it can employ chronic infections in the kidney and liver to increase scarring or it can use scarring to increase risk for infections. In the brain and heart, it employs thrombosis and the hypoxic-ischemic venue to increase scarring, while scarring can also increase risk for infections and seizures. What they have in common is that they utilize the full complement of immune arsenal and mesenchymal cells that they have at their disposal within interstitial spaces to activate venues. This has occurred because of the pervious effects of chronic inflammation on disabling the capillary cell dance and pirating their outer membranes.

Central to fibrous scar formation are duped mesenchymal cells that have switched allegiance to the anti-organ and begins secreting fibrous scar tissue or amyloid into the interstitial space. The scar tissue, not only take the place of atrophied end organ tissue, but further separates it from its oxygen source, the disabled capillary cell. This has the effect of slow asphyxiation of the end organ.

Can scarring be stopped or even reversed? Stem cells may provide answers but in the meantime aggressive reduction of vascular inflammatory free radicals may actually have the same effect as doing so removes the rust off the capillary cell pivot and swing dance to eventually stem and pace capillary cell, interstitial space and end organ recovery. This kind of thinking was not even imaginable just a decade ago. But then again, in a disease treatment models, it wouldn't be.

Scarring by its nature is a late effect of chronic inflammation. This makes scar reversal difficult and in some clinical realms not possible. If and when it does occur, it could potentially resuscitate multiple end organs as capillary cell find life in their dance footing. As might be expected, fatigue and pain remit as multiple chronic afflictions improve from a positive multi-end organ response.

As previously implied, scarring invites other anti-organ venues such as infections or cancer, thereby further perpetuating rapid end organ declines. In these setting, with the capillary cell and interstitial space already compromised, scarring can enable the systemic blood stream spread of cancer cells or infectious agents throughout the body. This is because scarring enables infectious agents and cancer cells to hide, grow and multiply, and then move their way through the harmless capillary cell into the blood stream, and elsewhere. In this fashion, scarring promotes metastasis of infections and cancer cells.

Fibrous scar tissue, amyloid, and tau represent a common venue employed by the anti-organ to further asphyxiate the end organ. Scarring can also be employed as a gateway to other anti-organ venues. In any event, it represents a late outcome to chronic inflammation and as such becomes very difficult to reverse if at all. Better to prevent than attempt to treat. Welcome to wellness.

Cancer

As difficult as it is for capillary and end-organ cells to come to terms with chronic inflammation within the interstitial space, it gets even more complicated when the anti-organ employs the cancer venue.

In the everyday life of an end organ, epithelial cells wear out and usually are replaced. When they need replacement capillary cell utilize the immune arsenal and mesenchymal cells within the interstitial space to remove them. Sometimes, these cells can go rogue and become cancer cells, in which case they are again quickly removed by the immune arsenal.

With chronic interstitial space inflammation, immune surveillance within the interstitial space gets *distracted* by fake messages and inflammatory chaos which is part of the overall plan of the chronic inflammatory matrix. To confuse and disrupt the immune arsenal to a point where they actually take cues to from the inflammatory matrix. Add chronic scar tissue, thrombosis, infectious agents or autoimmune complexes to the interstitial space mix, and cancer cells can find footing, hide, grow and multiply without being noticed by the discombobulated immune arsenal. When cancer reaches a certain critical mass, it no longer needs to be shielded as it can now resist any weapon coming at it. Its intent conforms to that of the anti-organ, which is to continue punishing the end organ, thereby making the anti-organ preeminence more powerful.

The fuel that creates immune distraction is interstitial space chaos, in part created by a robust display of vascular inflammatory free radicals. From combinations of AGEs, LDL cholesterol, triglycerides, lipoprotein (a) [abbreviated lipo(a)], homocysteine, and/or other free radicals from alcohol, tobacco or drug toxins, chronic interstitial space inflammation has blocked the capillary cell dance, decapitated its infrastructure and pirated its outer membranes. That enables the anti-organ to fully utilize the interstitial space immune arsenal and mesenchymal cells to its own advantage, which includes ignoring the growth of cancer cells. It is in this context that cancer cells find a foothold. Yes, lifestyle choices to the extent that they increase all the aforementioned vascular inflammatory free radicals, directly correlate with the emergence of cancer.

As cancer cells grow into a mass, they produce their own sets of venues, strategic defenses and blood supply, all at the expense of the end organ. In this sense, like the anti-organ before it, cancer actually piggybacks the anti-organ to become a second rogue end organ. Although most cancer growth appears uneven and even disorganized, there growth characteristics are aggressive and become increasingly difficult to contain. At some point cancer cells bud from the enlarging mass, disperse into an interstitial space, and find their way into the bloodstream where they metastasize generally through venous channels.

It would seem logical to conclude that chronic inflammation that is fueled by vascular inflammatory free radicals could eventually cause the emergence of the anti –organ, with a venue that would include cancer growth. Chronic inflammation can open up cancer occurrences anywhere, making the reduction of vascular inflammatory free radicals a priority in preventing late outcome cancer.

Treatment of cancer with surgery, chemo and radiation becomes an expensive and ineffective Band-Aid unless reducing vascular inflammatory free-radicals is integrated into the treatment plan. This has been shows recently with medicines that lower vascular inflammatory free radical burden, such as aspirin, beta-blockers, metformin and statins, also lower cancer occurrence rates while improving cancer treatment outcomes. This would also certainly hold true for exercise, dietary, stress and sleep interventions.

So cancer risk escalates with any chronic proinflammatory behavior(s) and conversely decreases with anti-inflammatory behaviors. Of course getting started late in the game makes deferring the risk difficult. This is because of established anti-organ venues in a very disabled capillary cell –interstitial space complex. When it comes to vascular inflammatory free radicals management and cancer prevention, every behavior matters. The *nightly bowel of ice cream or the glass of sherry with a cigarette can be enough to tip the scale.*

Infection

Similar to the way in which cancer cells find traction, bacteria, viruses, and other infectious agents can also utilize immune distraction created by chronic inflammation to find viable access within the interstitial space while being ignored by duped immune arsenal. Like cancer cells, they too can hide in scar tissue and multiply without being bothered. Infectious agents can mask their growth in many ways, They can hide in scar tissue, they can form their own microcosm (abscess), or in the case of viruses, can actually incorporate into the end organ cell's DNA or RNA. They can adapt their DNA on the fly to develop resistance to different antibiotic treatments, particularly if under dosed or if already resistant to their effects. This means chronic inflammation can afford infectious agents multiple opportunities to grow, multiply and disseminate. This eventually can result in invasion of the blood stream to metastasize elsewhere.

The presence of chronic inflammation and the anti-organ, when coupled by any of its other venues, doubles down the risk for interstitial space infection. In other words, the anti-organ venues both self-perpetuate and propagate different other venues that further coopt the interstitial space and destroy the end organ. All of them are fueled by vascular inflammatory free radicals.

As such, when chronic inflammation is connected to recurrent and chronic infections within the interstitial space it becomes another anti-organ white flag. Taking antibiotics or antiviral treatments can suppress or at times eliminate infectious symptoms. Unfortunately the nature of chronic inflammation and the disabled interstitial space usually allows for a return or recurrent infection. With chronic inflammation infectious treatment may stalemate the infection but eradication often becomes very difficult when other anti-organ venues, such as scarring or hypoxic-ischemia are compounding treatment.

Just like with scarring and cancer, chronic or recurrent infections that involve the anti-organ are late occurrences to an already compromised interstitial space and end organ. Reducing vascular inflammatory free radicals can produce some benefit, but the fact is that it is a long way back for the capillary cell to find footing and retool its dance so that it can effectively support enough immune recognizance to reverse recurrent or chronic interstitial space infection.

Autoimmune Disease

The anti-organ finds employment of rogue immunoglobulins a perfect fit to yet another venue that works against an already failing interstitials space and end organ. In this case, creating enough chaos within the interstitial space, coupled with the transitioning of the immune arsenal including immunoglobulins to a different boss, pressures immunoglobulin proteins within the interstitial space to seize and attach to proteins on membrane surfaces that belong to the end organ, members of the immune arsenal, or capillary cells. The autoimmune complex (also known as an antigen-antibody complex) once formed plumes additional inflammation towards it that includes white blood cells and cytokines. This deployment not only destroys the autoimmune complex but induces chain- reactions of countless other immunoglobulin attachments to expand the attack on the end organ's surface proteins and infrastructure. The very proinflammatory chain reaction is like a series of cluster bombs to the integrity of end organ outer membranes that perpetuate and accelerate end organ declines. The implementation of rogue immunoglobulins is a very effective venue as it causes a direct hit on the end organ as well as stir up inflammatory chaos in the interstitial space. This venue can be a cause or effect of other anti-organ venues that include scarring, thrombosis, infections and cancer.

Just like with other anti-organ venues, the induction of rogue immunoglobulins is fueled by chronic festering of vascular inflammatory free radicals. It is this perpetuation that has provided impetus for the prior pirating of capillary cell outer membranes by the inflammatory matrix that enables the anti-organ venues.

Of course, as rogue autoimmune carpet bombing continues on the end organ, it breeds escalation of other venues, just like other venues provide impetus for rogue immunoglobulins thereby self -perpetuating the anti-organ strategy. Rogue immunoglobulins create venues for scarring and cancer and visa- versa. As end organs fail, waves of chronic fatigue and pain increase dramatically. Disease treatment, while often heroic and sometimes lifesaving at this stage, is fraught with complications and other cascading risks. The autoimmune white flag has been raised.

Clearly, wellness is the best method to prevent rogue immunoglobulins or at least blunt their inflammatory margins before they carpet bomb. They key again involves creating enough anti-inflammatory impetus within the interstitial spaces to enable capillary cells to fight off the dance rust and begin to flux their outer membranes. This road is much easier to implement early rather than late in the game, when the anti-organ has fully retooled the interstitial space to its own liking. Nevertheless, when it comes to rogue autoimmune complexes, going all in to reducing proinflammatory behaviors can make a big difference in some cases, even late in the game. It certainly is worth a shot and makes other autoimmune treatments work better. This same principle can be used in fighting off other anti-organ venues that involve cancer or thrombosis. Even late in the game, anti-inflammatory lifestyles make more traditional disease treatments more effective.

Hypoxia and Ischemia

Thrombosis, or the process that induces blood to clot, in the wrong hands can induce hypoxic-ischemic events. Thrombosis, unless linked to trauma or injury, *never* benefits the involved end organ and usually translates into blood flow cutoff, oxygen asphyxiation, loss of end organ cells and subsequent decline in function. When it comes to thrombosis, both downstream larger vessel endothelial and upstream capillaries co participate in the escalation of sequential hypoxia to the end organ. The anti-organ uses the thickened and inflamed endothelial and capillary cell basement membranes to block its relationship with adjoining smooth muscle. Not only does the thickened and inflamed basement membrane limit access to adjoining smooth muscle, but is also applies stiffness to the lumen diameter to restrict blood flow through it. This becomes the catch that leads to hypoxic ischemic events upstream, as endothelial cells are rendered helpless to increase blood flow north and capillary cells are unable to match increased end organ oxygen demand to increased blood flow. The double whammy causes increases in interstitial space inflammation as end organ cells fight to prevent asphyxiation. As they atrophy or die, often insidiously rather than in mass, the anti-organ will again use other venues to supplement the thrombosis effect. These include getting mesenchymal cells to lay down scar tissue and amyloid to replace the loss of end organ volumes. Scarring can become a nidus for cancer, infection or rogue immunoglobulins.

Whereas, all of the inflammatory chaos is occurring within the interstitial spaces of the vascular tree, the actual clotting or thrombosis occurs within the lumens of the affected blood vessel(s) (see appendix, figure 18). In some cases, basement membrane plaque can rupture and spew inflammatory debris in all directions leading to a thrombosis. In other instances, pieces of clot can break off from inside the affected lumen, thrombose within the circulation, and lodge into a smaller upstream vessel to cause thrombosis and occlusion there. No matter where occlusions occur, and no matter what end organ is involved, they cut off blood flow, cause oxygen debt and asphyxiate the end organ.

The process of getting to a thrombosis can be just as unnerving to upstream capillaries as the thrombosis itself, as they do everything possible to try and support end organ screams for more oxygen. There efforts become increasing blunted as the end organ assumes control of the interstitial space and lays out the hypoxic-ischemic venue.

As mentioned thrombosis can disturb any end organ but is downright ruthless to the brain or heart. Whether from one large event or a stuttering of smaller events, thrombosis can leave their mark either as a cardiac cripple, with severe exertional breathlessness form heart failure, or in the form of various dementias linked to drooling, incontinence, a wheelchair and total absence of previous essence.

So, thrombosis is part of a joint effort employed by the anti-organ to occlude downstream lumens to cause hypoxic chaos in upstream interstitial spaces involving already disabled capillaries and their end organ partners. As the end organ asphyxiates, they are replaced by scar tissue, which can then breed other anti-organ venues that relentlessly dismantle what is left of the end organ. Just like other anti-organ venues, thrombosis is a late chronic inflammatory event linked to advancing endothelial and capillary cell basement membrane thickening from the accumulation of chronic vascular inflammatory free radicals. Blocking thrombosis chain reactions at this late stage can be difficult but reducing vascular inflammatory free radicals can decrease the pressure to further thicken endothelial and capillary cell basement membranes. Even when late in the game, there could be clinical utility in saving the brain or heart from progressive dementia or heart failure.

Thrombosis becomes another end organ white flag used by the

anti-organ as it takes advantage of the pirated capillary cell outer membranes and hypoxic conditions within the interstitial space. In the brain thrombosis involving small or large vessels completely disrupts function, induces cerebral atrophy and amyloid scarring to yield a stubborn progression of different dementias. In the heart, there is stunning loss of energy and the ability to mobilize, even from a chair. Neither of these late end organ outcomes makes life even remotely livable, but is exactly the impetus that breeds more disease treatment. We try hard to extend the lives of those that can barely think or walk but almost pay no attention reversing the chronic inflammation that pushed the process. Wellness please!

Conclusion

The goal of the anti-organ is to parlay the control of the capillary cell outer membranes and compromised interstitial space to develop venues that further isolate and destroy the end organ. This could be considered a late consequence of chronic inflammation, the final stage if you will. These venues would be considered white flags to end organ function as they often cause such a deep whole to climb out of that any return of end organ function becomes almost irrevocable. Anti-organ venues require a completely pirated and submissive capillary cell outer membrane to enable the anti-organ to bring what it wants from the blood plasma. It also requires that immune arsenal and mesenchymal cells within the interstitial space acquire a different play book that has been written by the anti-organ. This becomes critical as the anti-organ richly employs both in the execution of its venues.

The playbook utilizes scarring, cancer, infections, rogue immunoglobulins and thrombosis to different degrees and emphasis depending on what end organ is involved. One venue tends to be a cause or an effect of others, all of which feeds momentum of end organ destruction. All of these late machinations of chronic inflammation produce a plethora of different diseases that fuel traditional disease treatment models. Unfortunately being late in the game they require expensive interventions, are plagued with risky side effects, and breed more late game treatment antics. Quality of life outcomes to many of these late stage treatments are questionable.

This is opposed to wellness and prevention, which takes on chronic inflammation at a much earlier stage, when it can be tamed and where the anti-organ has not had a chance to evolve. The early stage resurrects the capillary cell dance by eliminating vascular inflammatory free radicals *before* anti-organ venues and diseases erupt.

The momentum against any of these sinister white flag outcomes requires intervention before there are symptoms. When choices are persistently good and are made early, the anti-organ is kept in isolation indefinitely. Keep the capillary cells dancing and white flags may never fly.

Chapter 7

TESTING FOR VASCULAR INFLAMMATION: THE HUNT FOR NITRIC OXIDE MEASUREMENT

Simple, direct and cost-effective measurement of the capillary-cell flux in outer membrane permeability is currently not possible. However a direct reflection of the blocked capillary cell dance is the reduction of mitochondrial volumes. Measuring the capacity of capillary cell mitochondrial to combust nitric oxide becomes a reflection of capillary cell mitochondrial mass and hence an indirect indicator of how well they are dancing.

The capillary cell nitric oxide response to an ischemic stimulus can now be estimated by using a finger temperature probe and measuring the change in temperature response before and after an arm blood pressure cuff has blocked blood flow to the finger for three to five minutes. Blocked arm blood flow produces hypoxia from lack of oxygen. When the arm blood pressure cuff is released, blood flow returns. The rate of return to the finger temperature after the release of the arm cuff becomes an indirect way of determining capillary cell nitric oxide response. How robust the nitric oxide response is becomes a reflection of capillary cell mitochondrial volumes, which then reflects the capillary cell dance.

With chronic inflammation within the interstitial spaces of end organs, the finger temperature response from a hypoxic stimulus sharply decreases. This test becomes a proxy to understanding how chronic inflammation is impairing capillary cells before there are symptoms or even before disease states are identified. It prompts attention to root causes of inflammation, provides a narrative for earlier discussions about wellness and lifestyle, before disease treatments are required. Measuring the finger -tip temperature response after a hypoxic stimulus becomes a litmus test to the health of capillaries and interstitial spaces they protect.

In the absence of or in combination with a finger temperature probe, another method of estimating chronic inflammatory risk within interstitial spaces is through a maximum exercise stress test where METS (maximum metabolic equivalent) is estimated on the basis of intensity of exercise. When the actual exercise MET is compared to a *predicted* maximum exercise MET of a 25 year old of the same sex and height, an adjusted *aging coefficient* can be obtained. The closer the coefficient is to one, the less aging (chronic interstitial space inflammation) that has occurred. Said differently, for a given individual, the closer they can maximally exercise to what would be predicted at age 25, the less chronic inflammation has occurred within interstitial spaces and the greater the likelihood that capillaries are dancing rigorously.

Other clues regarding capillary cell health can be obtained from blood work and imaging studies. The advantages to blood work are that they can be evaluated serially, can be relatively inexpensive, and can be used to assess the benefits of lifestyle, medicinal or supplement interventions. *Serial sampling,* perhaps every four to six months of targeted abnormal results can produce real time assessments of whether interventions are having anti-inflammatory benefits. In the grand scheme, serial blood measurements are an inexpensive snap shot and can further pique adjustments to anti-inflammatory routines and treatments. With resolve, lifestyle will not only reduce unwanted pounds, blood sugars, LDL cholesterol and blood pressures, but could also create less dependency on drug interventions. Let's start with what blood work to look at.

Blood Work

Initial blood screening should be fasting in the morning (no food after midnight prior to the test), and should include the following:

- **Complete blood count (CBC),** which includes testing for *hemoglobin, hematocrit, red* and *white blood cell* counts, and *platelet* counts; the CBC checks for *anemia,* which is often caused by iron deficiency, bone marrow problems, possible infection, and bleeding tendencies.

- **Comprehensive metabolic panel,** which includes *blood sugar, electrolytes,* and *liver* and *kidney function* tests. This basic blood work helps identify many evolving or preexisting proinflammatory conditions. As such it is fundamental to any screening evaluation and produces the biggest bang for the medical buck.

- **Hemoglobin A1C (HbA1C),** which is a sensitive marker of blood sugar control. This number increases with age and triggers a red flag when it exceeds 5.6. When it hits 6.5 diabetes is diagnosed.

- **Urine analysis,** to check for the presence of bacteria, white or red blood cells and protein.

- In selected cases, measuring **homocysteine** and **lipo (a)** levels, both of which can seed interstitial spaces as vascular inflammatory free radicals.

- Measuring levels of **magnesium, iron,** and **vitamins D** and **B$_{12}$,** all of which can decrease with advancing age.

- Measuring levels of **TSH, T3, and T4,** all of which together assess thyroid function and often decrease sequentially with aging.

- Measuring **LDL and HDL cholesterol levels** (and if possible, their particle size), **triglycerides,** and **highly sensitive C-reactive protein (HS-CRP).** HS-CRP provides a very useful snapshot of vascular inflammation and can be followed serially to determine effectiveness of anti-inflammatory treatments.

- In selected cases, hormone levels may need to be tested, including **cortisol, testosterone, estrogen,** and **progesterone**.

Ideally, treatment strategies should be reworked until inflammatory markers have normalized. There are no excuses for failing to do fasting blood work, as blood sampling is generally easy to collect and yields substantial clues about chronic inflammation.

Imaging and Stress Testing

Noninvasive imaging studies, either performed on a one-time basis or occasionally on a serial basis, can be useful in providing snapshots of large-vessel vascular disease and thereby an approximation of overall endothelial-cell inflammatory health. Examples of noninvasive imaging include:

Carotid duplex scans are noninvasive, relatively inexpensive ultrasound screening tests that assess large-vessel vascular disease in the 6 large arteries in the neck that supply 100% of blood flow to the brain. These tests, when initially abnormal, can produce a sense of urgency to medical anti-inflammatory intervention. They can be performed serially, without risk of contrast dye or radiation exposure, to assess plaque progression, and can also be used as a proxy for estimating large-vessel vascular disease elsewhere. Similarly, a one-time ultrasound assessment of the *abdominal aorta* can be lifesaving in assessing the risk for an expanding *abdominal aortic aneurysm.*

Exercise stress testing with ultrasound (*2-D or 3-D echocardiogram*), or *nuclear imaging,* can be helpful when routine stress testing produces an equivocal result. These tests are usually recommended when there is a high index of suspicion for symptomatic coronary artery disease. It can also be used to visualize leaking heart valves, estimate the extent of previous heart muscle damage, and to determine if heart muscle is at risk when exercised. In the absence of symptomatic coronary artery disease, this level of testing is generally not necessary.

The exercise stress test, in addition to establishing an aging coefficient, can be used to establish a safe exercise prescription and unmask serious heart-rhythm disturbances linked to exertion. A more detailed discussion about the exercise coefficient can be found in my first book, *Hazing Aging*.

Coronary calcium scores, magnetic resonance imaging (MRI), and *computerized tomography (CT) imaging* of the heart or carotid arteries, are generally not utilized serially because of their expense and lack of insurance coverage. They could be used on a one-time basis to accurately snap shot in those at high or known risk for preexisting vascular disease. The cost coupled with the duplication of information obtained from less expensive testing, limits their clinical utility. As such, they should be considered niche tests and utilized when other testing has yielded ambiguous results or the complexity of the clinical situation merits a more detailed view.

For best results, tests to assess vascular inflammation should be targeted and directly linked to treatment strategies where improvement can be verified and serially measured. In other words, unless a serial test result can be coupled to a treatment change, it should probably not be performed.

Conclusion

Inflammatory testing should be a way of determining chronic interstitial space inflammation before it has caused disease. The best methods couple evaluations that measure how well the capillary cells are dancing, with known vascular inflammatory free radical triggers. Winning the battle requires accurate surveillance of interstitial space hygiene, which involves the capillary pivot and swing dance, and until recently has not had any capability of being measured. Serial blood testing is valuable in that it provides measuring changes in vascular inflammatory free radicals and helps determine whether lifestyle, medications or supplements have made a difference or need further adjustment. The goal should be to catch inflammation before it catches us.

Chapter 8

THERAPEUTICS: REBALANCING CAPILLARY-CELL MITOCHONDRIAL ENERGY AND NITRIC OXIDE PRODUCTION

The goal of *wellness therapeutics* should be to restore the capillary-cell outer-membrane permeability pivot and mitochondrial combustion pendulum swing by ostensibly reducing end-organ interstitial-space vascular inflammatory free-radical seeds and subsequent immune arsenal plumes. When accomplished, the capillary cell dance is reset, rejuvenation returns to the capillary cell and its partners like a fountain of youth. This defines wellness as interstitial s pace hygiene is optimized and end organ function facilitated as chronic interstitial space inflammation does not get a curtain call. As long as capillary cells can dance, they promote integrity to the interstitial space and end organ. End organ function will surge, chronic illnesses get prevented, and fatigue and pain remit.

Capillary cells pace and stem rejuvenation on the feedback loop consciousness of their outer membranes and mitochondria. It is this unique interplay that not only improves each other's function but also that of its interstitial space partners the mesenchymal and end organ cells as well. All life depends on this endothelial and capillary flux. Dark influences will do everything within its power to block it.

The back and forth capillary cell pivot and swing dance is required to dual purpose capillary cell function. On the one hand, energy combustion supports active transport of immune arsenal into the interstitial space to mitigate inflammatory breach. When breach is mitigated, outer membrane permeability downshifts or pivots enabling mitochondrial combustion to swing from energy to nitric oxide thereby pacing repair, replacement and mitosis of outer membranes, organelles, and telomeres to itself and mesenchymal brethren, while increasing blood flow (and end organ mitochondrial energy combustion)to improve end organ function. Pacing end organ rejuvenation occurs when the capillary cell pivots permeability and swings combustion in the opposite direction. The best of therapeutics facilitates the capillary cell pivot an d swing.

Reducing vascular inflammatory free radicals is the foundation for wellness therapeutics. Chronic inflammation is subverted, and the subsequent chain reactions leading to the inflammatory matrix and anti-organ prevented. To address preventative therapeutics certain assumptions about inflammation can no longer be ignored. First, there is no such thing as compartmentalizing inflammation. It does not do damage in one locale but in all interstitial spaces everywhere. Second, making proinflammatory decisions are not cancelled out by anti-inflammatory ones. Exercising does not cancel out harm from a cigarette, binge alcoholism, a sleepless night or a bowl of ice cream. Third, lifestyle choices are not soft therapeutics but should be viewed as medicine choices. When we intentionally make bad choices, it is like not taking medicine correctly. No longer should these choices be seen as negotiable, ignored or considered incidental. Rather they should be viewed as the horse in front of the cart that drives or blocks inflammation. In this sense, adding medicinals and supplements to lifestyle become the cart. Fourth, aging is linked to vitamin and antioxidant deficiencies which need to be supplemented. Failing to do so, puts organelles, membranes and DNA at risk for dysfunction and free radical oxidative stress. Fifth, medicinals are often prescribed to treat diseases that manifest from chronic inflammation. They are not a substitute for anti-inflammatory lifestyle adjustments, can often be decreased or eliminated when lifestyles permit so.

Sixth, many medicines that are prescribed are actually proinflammatory in that over time they increase chronic inflammation. As such when prescribed they should be used only for brief periods and then withdrawn. Members of the proinflammatory group include hormones, bisphosphonates, narcotics, acid blockers, antibiotics, diet pills, steroids, most brain stimulants, and even nonsteroidal anti-inflammatory medicines like ibuprofen. Several other medicine groups, such as certain antidepressant and antipsychotic drugs, may also be in this camp.

The hallmark of preventative therapeutics is to produce a relatively tidy end-organ interstitial space. This space between capillary and end organ cells is where inflammation takes seed. As such it's hygiene, or lack of it, becomes a direct reflection to the back and forth capillary cell pivot and swing dance and all the virtues that follow. Good health is driven by periodic personal assessment and behavioral adjustment. This requires an ongoing intentional radar surveillance that involves lifestyle and is coupled with thoughtful targeting of medications and supplements that address emerging medical conditions while preventing vitamin and antioxidant deficiencies. There really is no such thing as a one-size-fits-all prescription, except that what we do, how and what we eat, and the medicines and supplements we consume should have an anti-inflammatory purpose. If the goal is to get the capillary cell outer membranes and mitochondria to tango, let's get started!

Exercise

There is no longer any debate about exercise and how it creates cascades of anti-inflammatory benefits. Exercise produces metabolic pathways that reduce blood stream vascular inflammatory free radicals while legitimizing a more ideal circulating energy substrate that energizes the endothelial and capillary cell dance. The dual mechanism that exercise provides is unlike other lifestyle interventions and therefore produces chain reaction boosters towards rejuvenation while also sanitizing interstitial spaces of vascular free radical seeds. In this sense, unlike any other intervention, exercise turns back the hands of time.

Exercise causes increased skeletal and heart muscle demand for more oxygen and energy substrate, as they require both to increase mitochondrial energy production. The energy along with calcium ions are fed to the sliding acting-myosin filaments to cause muscles to contract faster and with more force. This provides the backdrop of skeletal muscle support that exercise requires enabling a persistent increase in workload.

When heart and skeletal muscle increase oxygen and energy substrate utilization, beneficial metabolic cascades affect endothelial and capillary cells elsewhere. In skeletal and heart muscle capillary cells have rigorously pivoted permeability and pendulum swung combustion to nitric oxide to support both increases in blood flow and rejuvenation of their infrastructure, mitochondria and outer membranes. As skeletal muscle soaks up pyruvate and fatty acids like a sponge to be utilized by their mitochondria for energy, the benefits cascade as glycogen and glycerol reserves in the liver and adipose are drained. When exercise is performed in the morning before eating a meal, it is mostly adipose glycerol that gets drained, thereby reducing fat stores and promoting weight loss.

By reducing glycogen and glycerol storage, less triglyceride, LDL cholesterol production and gluconeogenesis occurs in the liver and fat. This has a net effect of reducing blood sugars, triglyceride, LDL cholesterol levels and homocysteine, while increasing blood HDL cholesterol. This blend of anti-inflammatory change reduces insulin resistance in all cells while decreasing multiple circulating vascular inflammatory free radicals. What is more, the LDL cholesterol that is circulating tends to be the larger more buoyant less inflammatory particle. All of this anti-inflammatory momentum provides ample impetus for endothelia and capillary cells throughout the body to flux permeability and swing combustion.

Regular exercise, with a mix of aerobic (continuous movement) and anaerobic (intermittent more forceful movement) will cause skeletal muscle to increase both filament thickness and mitochondrial volumes. Doing so gives skeletal muscle greater capacity to perform as well as allowing it to consume more pyruvate and fatty acids to make energy, as long as the endothelia and capillary cells can deliver ample blood flow. This discussion implies that regular and more rigorous exercise perhaps for 20-30 minutes produces unprecedented anti-inflammatory benefits that increase the capillary cell dance, sanitize interstitial spaces, and rejuvenate and augment end organ function while delegitimizing anti-organ intent on establishing proinflammatory venues.

Regular aerobic and anaerobic exercise becomes even more important as we age. Aging is associated with increased sarcopenia or loss of skeletal muscle mass (actin- myosin filament thickening) and tone (mitochondrial volumes), which increases insulin resistance and predilection for adult diabetes and additional waves of circulating vascular inflammatory free radicals. Regular exercise sharply reduces the insulin resistance and other vascular inflammatory free radical fall-out by preventing sarcopenia. Doing so also prevents falls and improves posture and gait. Exercise therefore becomes the gateway to wellness.

As expected, if exercise blocks chronic inflammation it also aggressively blocks anti-organ venues thereby preventing chronic and debilitating illnesses and their fatigue and pain fall-out. By decreasing diabetic risks exercise prevents its multiple proinflammatory complications. As weight is reduced blood pressure, blood sugars, LDL cholesterol and triglycerides decrease as well. As capillary cells dance at a pace years younger than expected, anticipated interstitial space chronic inflammatory outcomes take a back seat. The list of chronic inflammatory disease outcome improvements or remissions is increasing by the year but include reversal of sexual dysfunction, improvements is airway movement through the lungs, stabilized or improved memory and cognition, less depression, improved sleep, less perception of stress, improved stiffness and achiness in joints, and less breathlessness with exertion. This is on top of reductions in serious systemic infections, multiple different cancers, thrombotic- hypoxic-ischemic events, and different types of autoimmune complex diseases. All these benefits require a comprehensive approach to lifestyle that includes exercise. Exercising daily but smoking cigarettes or eating a large bowl of ice cream before bedtime will not get it done.

How to begin an exercise program is a major stumbling block for most people. Finding the time, motivation and the right kind of exercise can become major stumbling blocks. In addition, for best results, intensity of exercise must be addressed, which can be tricky with pre -existing medical problems. There not only is intensity of exercise a moving target that requires adjustment in either direction but training must also take into consideration age, sex, muscle mass, body mass index, arthritis pain, medical problems as well as heart or lung disease. Savvy personal trainers should be employed to help tailor and adjust the right kind and intensity of exercise. When in doubt about capacity to exercise a trainer's recommendation should be coupled with an exercise prescription from a health care provider. In these cases, a stress test may be a very useful screening tool to create a safe exercise prescription.

Exercise prescription for a given individual has a sweet spot, or a *therapeutic window of benefit*, based on the capacity to exercise. Capacity can improve as exercise improves heart and skeletal muscle conditioning must with aging and medical conditions, increased capacity must be managed with caution. Being able to exercise consistently, regardless of disability or preexisting medical conditions, should improve capacity. Conversely a medical set back, such as being admitted to the hospital for pneumonia, a surgery, or a broken bone can decrease capacity abruptly and more so with advanced age. Being able to adjust daily exercise, based on prevailing conditions involving our environment and physical capabilities, becomes a major determinant in exercise success. This would imply that success requires a certain level of intuition about what we can do and why we do it. Exercise prescription, therefore, is fluid, and will need adjustments based on improvement in exercise tone or alternatively reduced in periods of surgical recovery or evolving medical conditions.

Daily aerobic exercise (walking, jogging, hiking, swimming, elliptical, treadmill, stationary biking, cycling, or rowing) for at least twenty to twenty five consecutive minutes, reduces chronic inflammation in interstitial spaces of all end organs. Ideally, it should also include at least 5-10 minutes of daily *anaerobic* (weight-lifting) movement of different large muscle groups. The fit and finish of exercise, particularly in those over 50 years of age, is completed by a few minutes of stretching and balancing. A pragmatic approach would consist of twenty-twenty five minutes of aerobic exercise, five to ten minutes of light weight lifting, and about five minutes of stretching and balancing. This amounts to 30-45 minutes of daily exercise or less than one hour in a 24 hour period.

Advanced aerobic training, while not for everyone, could have further anti-inflammatory and anti-aging benefits. It usually involves *intervals of intense aerobic exercise*, where heart and breathing rates are at close to maximal effort, followed by periods of less effort. Interval training, as well as other extreme types of exercise (for example, marathon-triathlon training or heavy weight lifting) can be dangerous in those with advanced age or with multiple medical conditions. Participation could lead to serious muscle or joint injury, heart attacks, asthma, dizziness, syncope or even sudden death. Extreme exercise should be performed only by those who are well conditioned, have been advised by a health care provider to do so, and are well versed with understanding attendant risks.

Lifting weights should not be a chore. Ideally it should complement an aerobic workout, and include 1-3 sets of between 12-20 repetitions of alternating large muscle groups to produce the best results. This could include something as simple as squatting (with or without weights), flat or upright bench presses and push-ups. To avoid injury, weight lifting should always be done with proper technique, which implies a slower and full range of motion. With advanced age or when exercising alone, weight machines are safer than free weights as they help control balance. The key principles about weight training should always involve *safety* first, erring on the side of *lifting lighter*, and following a program suitable for each individual's body habitus and preexisting medical conditions.

With aging, posture, gait and balance mechanics suffer, and coincide with tendencies for tendons, muscles, and ligaments to become painful and stiff, and for bones to become soft or brittle. These changes make exercise more difficult and therefore mandate a modified exercise prescription. Obesity, previous injury, or chronic pain can worsen pain from certain exercise movements thereby requiring adjustment and a "go slow" exercise policy. Although challenging, physical disabilities should not veto an exercise program. If achiness becomes overwhelming, exercise should be stopped and the hunt for the cause of the pain should be addressed.

Stretching, even for just a few minutes, becomes more important with advanced age, as stiffness reduces full range of motion to many joints and muscles. This cascades to effect posture and gait, which then increases risk for falls and fractures. Stretching helps counterbalance muscle and joint stiffness. *Balance exercises* can also protect against falls. Breaking long bones or compressing a lumbar vertebra because of falling produces serious and sometimes extended or permanent disability, and could be prevented by a few minutes of daily stretching and balancing.

The keys to a successful exercise program are commitment, adapting to a physical injury or medical condition, and finding the time to do it consistently. Developing *alternative* exercise strategies, while *anticipating* exercise limitations before they occur, can go a long way in making *adjustments* to maintain a regular exercise program.

Exercise is a mindset. It finds opportunity when time or circumstances don't work in its favor. For example taking the stairs instead of an elevator, walking 6 blocks to a destination instead of hailing a cab, or doing a set of push-ups or squats in a hotel room before showering, all contribute to exercise equivalents. Morning exercise before breakfast, burns more fatty acids, and therefore is a great way to kick start weight loss. Tweaking intensity can make exercise more effective, but in those over 45 years of age or with medical problems, must be done with a sobering assessment of risk and benefit. When in doubt, exercise stress testing can result in a safe exercise prescription.

Summary

Regular exercise is a pluripotent modifier to chronic interstitial-space inflammation. By decreasing multiple vascular inflammatory free radicals while optimizing energy substrate to all cells, it produces potent anti-inflammatory momentum that centers on the pivot and swinging of the capillary cell dance. By facilitating the endothelial-capillary cell dance, exercise helps to sanitize the interstitial space, rejuvenate endothelia and capillary cells and their partners, and improve end organ function. All anti-organ chronic inflammatory venues decrease including different cancers, heart conditions, dementia and disabling arthritis. Pain and fatigue diminish to the extent we can exercise. Hello *Rejuvenation!*

Nutrition

Food is medicine and medicine is food. It can work for us or create such inflammatory momentum that it can destroy us. It is something that we all require to survive, often take for granted with our choices decided by a complex array of old habits, addictions taste and texture preference, and in some cases, deceptive information. Many of the reasons why we buy certain food and beverages are misguided.

Besides the obvious, foods that are high in sugars and trans-fats, we can make choices in a grocery store that we think are good, but are actually bad. This is because labeling does not tell the complete story. Labels can hide certain sugars, trans-fats and even lack full disclosure about chemical sprays, hormones, growth stimulants and engineered genetic modifications. This means, off the shelf, unlike electronics for example, we really don't know what composes the product we are buying. So, even when we are well intentioned, when it comes to food choices, it's often is a crap shoot.

It doesn't have to be this way, but in the name of profit, improved efficiency, taste, safety, shelf life and labeling misconceptions, it has become much harder, not easier to buy quality food. Modern nutrition has become a contentious topic, as a growing chorus of decent would say these benefits have come at too much of an expense to quality and in some cases, safety.

As food has become more engineered and processed, the risk for transmitted infections have decreased, but the end product often contains empty sugar calories, very little fiber and lost vitamins and minerals. The trade of processed for unprocessed foods has reduced infectious transmissions but has produced an epidemic of sugar and salt laced addicting fast and prepackaged foods that have escalated alarming rates of obesity, hypertension, adult diabetes, the metabolic syndrome and all the inflammatory fallout that follows. Even more sinister is what this food can cause down the line. Dementia, disabling arthritis, heart disease, numerous cancers and autoimmune disorders are just a few outcomes. Understanding the long term risk of these foods to our health has just barely scratched the surface.

Three misconceptions about food have bred this firestorm and deserve mentioning. First, the concept that *all calories are created equal* has co-opted food engineering, making simple sugar calories found in an energy bar equivalent to the complex carbohydrate calories found in kale or spinach. The falsehood implies that it does not matter where calories come from; it is just about the total calories ingested. This makes it okay to eat whatever you want or substitute at will say an energy bar for a salad on the basis that the body will take whatever calories it gets from either source and use them wisely. Total calories are more important than where they come from.

A second misconception is that all fats are bad. It turns out eating a certain amount of fat is vital to our health, but not all fats are created equal when it comes to inflammation. Although there is still much to learned about fat metabolism, it is clear that ingesting monounsaturated oils, such as avocado or olive oil, coupled with omega three oils found in fatty fish, nuts and flax produce anti-inflammatory benefits when eaten regularly and in modest quantities. Even some saturated fats when consumed in small quantities and from non - animal sources, may be beneficial to our health.

The third major nutrition snafu is that engineering food to increase harvest or to resist insects has no material impact on its quality. While the jury may still be out on genetic modifications and the harm they potentially cause, it would only make sense that a genetically engineered apples twice the size of the original and with substantial increases in sugar content, would have less nutritious benefit compared to the original. It goes without saying that the chemical sprays and hormones that are quietly used to increase yields and prevent infection also have their own set of hidden risks that we look the other way to. Can you see why buying food can get bizarre? It would seem that the more we know, the more we don't know about what we buy.

One thing about food is clear. Whole, natural, unprocessed food is better than purchasing the sum of its parts. And plant food has the best complement of vitamins, minerals, fiber and nutrient compared to other sources. Whether from edible tubers, roots, flowers, leaves, seeds, or fruit, the combinations of them provide a blend of nutrient-rich fiber, protein, antioxidants, vitamins, and healthy fats, which in aggregate, block chronic inflammation through a variety of different cellular mechanics. Diets rich in natural plant fiber, improves the constituency of bacteria that make up the intestinal microbiome. With a better bacterial population within the intestinal lumen, the tone it set for improved nutrient absorption. Not only do more minerals and antioxidants get absorbed, but simple sugars *trickle* rather than *rush* to the liver after being absorbed. Trickling changes the entire dynamic of how the liver sinusoid manages glycogen storage, how much and what type of energy substrate it ships to adipose cells, LDL cholesterol production, and most important, how much blood sugar is circulating throughout the body.

Modern food processing not only eliminates vitamins, minerals and fiber, but often adds back salt, sugars and preservatives to improve taste and increase shelf life. Sometimes they are fried or baked in polyunsaturated vegetable oils which quickly turn to trans-fats when heated. The prepackaged combinations can be very tasty, but the sugar, salt and trans-fat make them very addictive and proinflammatory. The combination of sugar, salt and trans-fat, when consumed regularly, will increase blood pressure (shear), blood sugars, and LDL cholesterol.

This deadly trio salt, sugar, and trans–fats are overproduced and underreported in most prepackaged labeling. The biggest offenders are cold meats, chips, crackers, cereals, breads, cookies, and desserts. Other offenders include off the shelf yogurt, ice cream, coffee creamers, fruit juices and colas.

Not only are trans-fats underreported, but so are sugars. Sugars other than sucrose (table sugar) may not be reported as sugar. This means that simple sugars such as lactose (found in diary), fructose (found in fructose corn syrup), sorbitol, and alcohol sugars may not be counted as sugars. Substitution of sugars and artificial flavors is common for example in the maple syrup industry. The cost of selling pure maple syrup would be unappealing to most. By making the syrup with artificial flavor and fructose coru syrup, the cost goes down ten- fold, but the increased inflammation caused from fructose and artificial preservatives goes up by about as much. Food labeling has been rigged to make foods appear less risky by hiding sugars and trans-fats according to the law. Over time, chronic inflammation stakes out interstitial spaces, disables the capillary cell dance, enables the anti-organ venues with dementia, cancers, infections, autoimmune diseases and crippling arthritis establishing firm footholds.

We I talk about vegetables, I am referring primarily to green leafy or cruciferous varieties. They include a staple of broccoli, kale, chard, spinach, cabbage, asparagus, cauliflower, Brussel sprouts and onion. If eaten whole, fresh and slightly cooked, they afford the best opportunity for optimizing nutrient presentation to the liver. This translates into better nutrient- absorption mechanics, fewer circulating vascular inflammatory free radicals, and a happier endothelial-capillary cell.

Making cruciferous vegetables a staple can circumvent acquired or inherited sensitivities to *gluten* (a protein found in grains) and *lactose* (a simple sugar found in dairy products). These two constituents can contribute to varying degrees of bloating, abdominal cramps, nausea, and diarrhea which can worsen as we get older. These sensitivities behoove a dietary bias towards more plant fiber.

Over the last fifty to sixty years, fad diets that scam rapid weight loss have invaded the landscape. These diets often cause rapid weight loss from dehydration or from forcing the liver to manufacture ketones to be used as energy substrate rather than glucose or fatty acids. This result is more metabolic stress and yo-yoing of weight loss and gain. The extreme metabolic bounces that these diets cause increase risks for large fluctuations in blood sugars increasing risks for more inflammation. Adding in diet pills or stimulants only makes yo-yoing and metabolic fluctuation worse. Couple yo-yoing weight with diet pills will increase heart palpitations, pulmonary hypertension, nervous and emotional irritability, sleep deprivation, psychosis and even sudden death.

A healthy diet, even for weight loss, does not involve fads of extremes. Food should be whole, as much plant based as possible, and should not be contaminated with pesticides, hormones, heavy metals (mercury, aluminum, or arsenic), or other toxins. The ideal diet should contain fresh vegetables, mixed proteins, and *monounsaturated and omega-3 oils*. The following list summarizes an optimal diet plan for most adults:

- **Protein.** About 45–60 grams of protein should be consumed daily, from a mix of fresh vegetables, fresh wild fish, free-range poultry, mixed nuts, unprocessed cheese (if not lactose intolerant), organic free-range eggs, and mixed beans. Those recovering from injury, operation or wound healing, or rigorously exercising, may require more protein, up to 80 grams (or more) daily. The capacity to process larger amounts of protein is dependent on competent kidney and liver function.
- **Complex Carbohydrates.** An abundant and diverse volume of complex carbohydrates from plant fiber, including fresh cruciferous vegetables, leaves, legumes, sprouts, edible roots,

and herbs. Simple *mono-* and *disaccharide* sugars should be restricted. This would include all simple sugars from fruit juices, colas, other soft drinks, desserts, white-flour products, white rice, and artificial sugar substitutes. Because of its abundant sugar content, fruit should be restricted to two servings daily, with most berries and grapes preferred. Because sugar is addicting, often under-labeled, does not reduce hunger, and does not necessarily taste sweet, it is ubiquitous in highly processed foods and directly contributes to obesity, diabetes and the metabolic syndrome. Sugar substitutes can be as bad, or even worse, than sugar itself! Whole grains and white rice are not really "whole" but rather mostly refined sugar and should be avoided. Steel cut oats are an exception.

- **Fats.** If weight loss is a goal, fat consumption should be limited but *not* avoided. In any case, fats should be primarily *monounsaturated oils,* such as olive, avocado, or coconut oil, and *omega-3 fatty acids* from flaxseed, nuts, and fish. Fried and breaded food, saturated fat from organ and red meats, and *polyunsaturated* vegetable-fat oils, particularly when used to cook with, should be avoided. With polyunsaturated vegetable oils (corn, canola, safflower, peanut oils), heat easily converts them to trans-fats.

- **Fluids.** In those without heart, liver or kidney failure, water consumption of about two liters (quarts) per day is recommended. For those rigorously exercising or working in hot and humid conditions, drinking more water will be required. Tea and coffee consumption in moderation (one to two cups per day of each) can help reduce all kinds of chronic inflammation. All colas, soft drinks, and fruit juices should be avoided or severely restricted. Milk can be associated with both lactose and protein intolerances. The nonfat varieties should be avoided as they harbor too much sugar. The risk- benefit ratio of alcohol works against us as we age and should mostly be avoided. If alcohol is ingested at all, red wine at 3 ounces every other day for men and every day or less for women is all that can be endorsed.

Although these recommendations apply for most adults, there will be exceptions based on food sensitivities and intolerances. In addition to the well- recognized gluten and lactose intolerances, other foods that produce sensitivities include protein allergies from eggs, certain meats, peanuts, and shellfish. In those who have been diagnosed with inflammatory colitis, ileitis, or other autoimmune gastrointestinal disorders, an even more restricted dietary spectrum may be required.

Other recommendations are linked to contaminated water from oceans, streams or lakes. Contamination from ocean fish is usually from mercury. Fresh water fish could harbor pesticides or residues from toxic farm fertilizer runoff. The safest bet is to eat fish 1-2 times per week, preferably caught wild, and with abundant omega three fatty acids, found in salmon, tuna, and mackerel.

Other recommendations that benefit reductions in chronic inflammation include eating one small piece (one inch square) of 60–70 percent (or higher) dark chocolate daily and eating eggs, meat or poultry that is free range, and fed without hormones. Nuts should be mixed without salt or roasted. If possible, food should not be microwaved. Cooking should be on low or medium heat and for less than 20 minutes. Burning or singeing meat or vegetables on high heat should be avoided. Salad dressing should be kept simple with combinations of olive oil, lemon, vinegar and herbs.

Cultivating a vegetable-herb garden should be on everyone's to-do list. The garden should include a selection of dark-green, purple, and/ or red cruciferous or leafy vegetables and an assortment of herbs. Gardening can be fun, but there is a learning curve, and there may be some failures early on. Everyone can develop a green thumb, but it requires practice. Getting some seasoned help (no pun intended) in the early stages of gardening can make the process more successful.

When it comes to food safety, short of growing your own, you simply have to hedge your bets. Fresh wild fish will likely have small amounts of mercury in its flesh, while farm-bred fish could have pesticides, antibiotics, and/or hormones in theirs. Likewise, farm-bred poultry, beef, and pork may have their growth stimulated by hormones, antibiotics, or appetite stimulants. GMO fruits and vegetables are engineered to grow faster and larger, but often with less nutrient value and more sugar. In many cases, pesticides have been used, food coloring added, and chemicals sprayed to delay spoilage and enhance appearance. Practically all snack foods, breads, and pasta have been produced with highly refined white flour, contain preservatives, and are baked or fried in oils that convert to inflammatory trans- fats. The combination of sugar, preservatives, trans- fat and salt produces major vascular inflammatory risks to the capillary cell dance. All of this is not meant to shock you but rather to serve as a reminder that buying food must be approached with a certain level of scrutiny. There is a learning curve but purchasing correctly does minimize vascular inflammatory free radicals which over time could contribute to the numerous venues of chronic inflammation.

Summary

By drinking large daily quantities of water, while eating fresh organic vegetables, herbs, beans, non- roasted or salted nuts, and dousing them with avocado or olive oil and fresh berries, provides the foundation for an anti-inflammatory diet. When combined with quality protein sources that include eggs, steel cut oats, non- processed cheese (for those not lactose intolerant), and free-range poultry and wild salmon, a well- diversified anti-inflammatory diet has been constructed that is both low glycemic and trans-fat. When purchasing food, have a high index of suspicion about hidden sugars, trans- fats, hormones and preservatives. Thoroughly wash all fresh fruit and vegetables after purchase. Try gardening fresh vegetables and herbs to diversity fresh produce. When a low salt, *glycemic*, and trans-fat diet is coupled with regular exercise, stress reduction, and improved sleep hygiene, the likelihood of chronic inflammation and anti-organ venues diminish, as the capillary cell dances and rejuvenates and paces vigor to the interstitial spaces and end organ it serves.

Stress and Sleep

Too much stress, too little sleep, or combinations of both, can chronically increase blood levels of *cortisol, adrenaline,* and *noradrenaline (catecholamine),* the so-called *stress hormones.* These hormones predispose to overheating and induce weight gain to increase insulin resistance and predispose to adult diabetes. In other words, persistent sleep deprivation and stress produce the opposite effect to our metabolism compared to regular exercise. In addition, stress and sleep deprivation induce dietary behaviors favoring the consumption of more junk food which cascades to accelerate weight gain, increase blood pressure, produce more anxiety and worsen depression. At the cellular level, capillary-cell pivot and swing dance becomes severely impaired, as the interstitial space organizes proinflammatory agendas. If allowed to continue, it becomes just a matter of time before the anti-organ unleashes its venues.

Stress and sleep deprivation increase vascular inflammatory free radical burdens within interstitial spaces by nurturing other malignant proinflammatory behaviors that include addictions or binges of alcohol, tobacco, drugs and sugars. All of these actually further perpetuate stress and sleep deprivation. In this manner, their proinflammatory menagerie produces an every widening circle of inflammation enabling to emergence within interstitial spaces of the chronic inflammatory matrix and anti-organ.

Sleep deprivation is not just caused from insomnia, not sleeping long enough or from addictions, but can also be triggered by frequent trips to the bathroom, a disturbing bed partner, daytime naps, variable work shifts, too much background noise, light, or obstructive sleep apnea. Stress almost always increases sleep deprivation and sleep deprivation will increase stress, hence they fuel and feed each other and co-contribute to maladaptive behaviors.

Stress is a *perception* about a conflict or predicament that produces a maladaptive emotional response that culminates in excessive anxiety or a depressed mood. Stress becomes a problem when the anxiety and depressed mood persists. It is often made worse with self- treatment utilizing alcohol, sugar, drugs or tobacco. In other words, stress and our attempts to mitigate often cascade poor judgement which culminates in behaviors that make the stress worse.

Because stress and sleep deprivation often precipitate poor coping choices interventions to mitigate them cannot be vague but specific and intentionally directed. Instead of saying "You should reduce stress," a better recommendation would be to say you should take a daily morning walk instead of having the donut with coffee. Maladaptive behaviors often link to increase stress and sleep deprivation. Going to a bar for a drink after work usually leads to either getting drunk, eating too much or other inappropriate behaviors. Instead, skip the bar routine and instead go to the gym and work out. Substituting bad behavior for good is a good way of mitigating stress and sleep deprivation. On occasion, stress and sleep deprivation are worsened from underlying medical conditions such as an overactive bladder, asthma, heartburn, thyroid conditions, sleep apneas or depression. All these conditions should be identified and treatment strategies initiated.

Effective treatment for stress and sleep deprivation requires a combination of disentangling medical problems, eliminating addictions and maladaptive behaviors, and making adjustments in the environment that are causing the stress or sleep deprivation. Treatment requires engagement and a sobering assessment of attendant risks and subsequent adjustments. Change will not come easy as complicated work- life situations coupled with addictions usually result in slip-ups or backsliding. Besides dissecting the stressful issue to find a resolution and paying attention to addictions, adding back in regular exercise, a healthy plant-based diet and a nurturing supportive environment that involves family and friends are also critically important.

Aging escalates the risk for increased stress, sleep deprivation and social isolation. Coupled with assorted chronic illnesses, multiple medications, and the reduced physical and mental capability to handle obligations, and it only makes sense that sleep deprivation and stress increase. It is not uncommon to forgo exercise, watch hours of daily television, forget or ignore prescription medications, drink alcohol before bedtime and eat only fast food. All of these behaviors potentiate stress and sleep deprivation. Making adjustments can get increasingly more difficult but to avoid a nursing home, diapers, dementia and dependency on others, there is no other choice.

Increases in stress and sleep deprivation, and the cascades of poor decisions they precipitate, perpetuate and accelerate chronic interstitial space inflammation. In the elderly this becomes a fast track to dementia, debilitating arthritis, falls, fractures, and infections.

Below are some important interventions that should improve sleep quality and mitigate stress as we age:

- Reduce financial and social obligations. Simplify decision making, Keep relationships simple. Reduce-eliminate conflict.
- Get help for things you cannot or no longer want to do.
- Stay independent for as long as you possibly can.
- Try to keep your own space and set your own pace.
- Do things that pique passion and provide joy.
- Try to read daily.
- Do everything you can to prevent falls-better lighting, easier access of walkways, use of rails, cane, walker etc.
- Try to exercise regularly.
- Eliminate caffeinated beverages after 2:00 p.m. Alcohol should be avoided. If consumed, it should not be within four hours of bedtime.
- Quiet the brain before sleep, with prayer, meditation, or selected reading that is not threatening or overly stimulating.
- Go to bed at the same time each night.
- Avoid frequent trips to the bathroom by limiting fluid intake for four hours before bedtime.
- Adjust/eliminate medicines that adversely affect sleep.

- Arthritis pain medicines (NSAIDS like aspirin, ibuprofen, or naproxen) can aggravate esophageal pain (GERD) and should be avoided before sleep.
- Limit napping during the day.
- Eliminate nighttime snacking or giving into insomnia by watching television, reading, or surfing the Internet.
- Sleep apnea should be treated, and other conditions that may contribute to anxiety or breathlessness at night should be addressed.
- Eliminate drug abuse, sugar addiction and tobacco use.
- If working, adjust work schedules if at all possible to reduce working different shifts or night shift work.

Summary

The management of stress and sleep deprivation is a moving target that becomes increasingly important as we age. This means we should not have as many "balls in the air" and those that we do, we enjoy. Both stress and sleep deprivation impair our coping skills as we make poor often addicting choices in attempts to mitigate, which only make the conditions worse. Recommendations for intervention should be specific and underlying medial conditions should also be summarily looked for and treated. For best results there should be a support structure in place that involves spouses, family, and friends. Support groups, such as alcoholics anonymous, can also be helpful in breaking addictions. Adding back in other anti-inflammatory behaviors, such as regular exercise, and plant based eating, are also helpful.

Stress and sleep deprivation compromise end organs by spiraling chronic interstitial inflammation. Eventually, they block the capillary cell pivot and swing dance, enable anti-organ interstitial space venues that cascade a litany of serious and often life-threatening illnesses. Getting an effective handle on stress and sleep deprivation often means the difference between living independently and living demented with wet diapers in a nursing home. What a difference less worry and uninterrupted sleep means to the final chapters of life.

Medicinals and Antioxidants

To menace chronic inflammation, medications and antioxidants (or vitamins) must do one of three things. They must either *reduce inflammatory-free radical burden* in the interstitial space, *increase antioxidant levels* and *metabolic cofactors,* or optimize *energy substrate ratios.* The first of these produces a direct hit on chronic inflammation, as vascular inflammatory free radicals, that fuel and perpetuate the spread of interstitial space inflammation, are decreased. By reducing them sufficiently, the rust comes off capillary cell's outer membranes, as they are enabled to downward flux permeability to subsequently swing mitochondrial combustion to nitric oxide, thereby initiating the capillary cell dance. Without reducing free radical concentrations within the interstitial space, the last two mechanisms *temporize* capillary cell function by optimizing the mitochondrial footprint without necessarily abetting the capillary cell dance.

In the grand scheme of chronic inflammation, medicines and supplements in themselves become relatively impotent if not coupled with a comprehensive anti-inflammatory lifestyle. Therefore, these therapies should be viewed as *complementary to, not exclusionary of,* chronic inflammatory treatment. Since medications and supplements improve capillary and endothelial cell mechanics in different ways, they often work even better when used in combination. Collectively and when combined with anti-inflammatory behaviors, their anti-inflammatory benefits provide enough momentum to block the stubborn overtures created by chronic interstitial-space inflammation.

It is postulated that medicinal and antioxidant anti-inflammatory mechanics facilitate the following:

- By reducing inflammatory free-radical burden within the interstitial space, they facilitate a capillary cell outer membranes bias towards reduced permeability to inflammatory mediators entering the interstitial space.
- As interstitial space free radicals decrease and capillary cell outer membrane permeability fluxes downward, mitochondria

pendulum swing combustion to nitric oxide. This increases blood flow to the capillary bed to push increases in end organ function, while also enabling capillary cells to rejuvenate. Pro clotting (thrombosis) mechanics simultaneously decrease.

- The capillary cell *stems and paces* similar infrastructure rejuvenation to its mesenchymal cell brethren within the interstitial space while reciprocating rejuvenation in end organ cells.
- The mechanics of rejuvenation involve many feedback loops and sub loops, but are created by the induction of capillary-cell *peroxisome proliferator receptor gamma coactivator (PGC-1-alpha)* and activation of mitochondrial nitric oxide synthetase.
- Rejuvenation induces among other things replication and replacement of capillary cell outer membrane receptors, mitochondrial volumes and lengthening of nuclear telomeres.
- Antioxidant levels increase, through combinations of increased production and decreased utilization caused by diversifying combustion free radical exhaust from the back and forth swinging of mitochondrial combustion. Antioxidants also increase through ingestion from supplements and improved nutrient.

By reducing vascular inflammatory free radical seeding of the interstitial space, medicinals produce a triple -*whammy effect* on chronic inflammation. This means the interstitial spaces of large arterial vessels downstream, as well as upstream capillaries are co enabled to improve their pivot and pendulum swing dance. This in turn co facilitates an improved working feedback loop relationship between them to nurture end organ supply oxygen and nutrient. The third rung of this improved downstream endothelial and-upstream capillary cell alliance is to expand improvement to the rest of the arterial vessel infrastructure and end organs. This expansion of anti-inflammatory benefit, to include the entire arterial circulation, facilitates across the board improvements in all end organs thereby establishing there wellness as the homeostasis bar is raised. The triple whammy effect involving endothelial, capillary and all end organ cells has been completed. Chronic inflammation is shut down everywhere and has no place to hide.

In some cases, medicinals, such as statins, can cause a dramatic reduction in vascular free radicals within interstitial spaces. This reversal can actually reverse basement membrane thickening and obstructive plaque development to further improve blood flow dynamics to upstream capillaries and end organs. Medicinals, such as metformin, help reset the glycolysis, gluconeogenesis and mitochondrial combustion relationship, which results in less insulin resistance and potentially less superoxide free radical exhaust from mitochondrial combustion.

In addition to downshifting gluconeogenesis and diverting fatty acid mitochondrial combustion towards pyruvate, medicinals and supplements can help facilitate mitochondrial acetyl CoA shuttling away from the Krebs cycle (energy combustion) and towards ribosomes or to the smooth endoplasmic reticulum outside of the mitochondria for protein synthesis. This acetyl CoA shuttle is a key component to rejuvenation that is induced by mitochondrial nitric oxide combustion. Finally, supplements can help improve the efficiency of either energy or nitric oxide combustion within mitochondria by augmenting necessary cofactors for electron transfer, increasing amino acid precursors utilized in nitric oxide production, or by facilitating antioxidant levels to help eliminate their free radical exhaust.

Age biases reduced capillary cell efficiency to affect interstitial space sanitation and respond to end organ oxygen demands. This is caused form combinations of accumulated DNA damage, chronic interstitial space inflammation, reduced intracellular antioxidants and decreased mitochondrial volumes. These combination of untoward events, unless addressed aggressively with intentional intervention puts a dagger into the guts of capillary cell functional mechanics. This is where medicinals and vitamin supplements work. They help fill I the gaps that have been caused by DNA misfires, reduced mitochondrial volumes and nitric oxide production, and fewer antioxidants. The hope is that capillary cells can still muster enough oomph to dance enough to stem the effects of chronic interstitial space inflammation.

Let's begin with the group that produces a direct assaults on chronic inflammation by removing one of its major fuel sources, the powerful small particle oxidized LDL cholesterol.

Statins, Niacin (Vitamin B$_3$), and Ezetimibe

Statins, niacin, ezetimibe, and a new class of medications known as the *PCSK9 inhibitors,* are medications that substantially reduce end-organ interstitial-space inflammation by reducing, a major vascular inflammatory free-radical seed, also known as *small-particle oxidized LDL cholesterol.* Small-particle (as opposed to the large, bulky-particle LDL cholesterol) oxidized LDL cholesterol (or LDL cholesterol) is a sticky, vascular inflammatory free radical that is produced in the liver, travels through the blood stream, easily migrates through the outer membranes of endothelial and capillary cells, to enter the interstitial space. Once in the interstitial space it globs onto membrane surfaces, including the capillary and endothelial cell basement membranes. Once they attach, if not promptly removed by an HDL particle, it acts almost as if it was an immune complex, attracting immune arsenal towards it. The pluming of inflammation, can over time, especially if accompanied by many more LDL particles, induces a chronic inflammatory response on the basement membrane.

This chronic inflammatory response thickens the basement membrane and makes it less responsive to the interstitial space, mesenchymal cells or the end organ. In larger vessels, intimal thickening stiffens the vessel thereby blocking surrounding smooth muscle overtures to expand the lumen diameter. This prevents adjustments in blood flow that are called for by upstream capillaries based on end organ demands. This is a strategic No- no to optimizing end organ and often generates SOS signals threatening upstream hypoxia-ischemia. With progression, intimal thickening can actually get worse to become an obstructive plaque. This usually causes upstream end organ desperation for more blood flow, which cannot occur. End organs such as brain nerve cells or heart muscle cells are tortured until they either severely atrophy or die. Different shades of dementia and heart failure are the outcomes based on what blood vessel is most besieged.

LDL cholesterol can create a sufficient chronic inflammatory blow to basement membranes to knock out the capillary cell dance. A persistent block of the endothelial and capillary cell pivot-pendulum swing dance becomes a recognizable first step that enables chronic interstitial space inflammation to form a matrix.

Small particle LDL cholesterol concentrations within the blood stream increase with age and are linked to genetic profiles, obesity, sugar ingestion, inactivity and hypertension. They can increase dramatically in post- menopausal women, suggesting a link to declining estrogen levels. Increases in blood plasma LDL cholesterol signals become a major red flag to interstitial space endothelial and capillary cell basement membrane thickening. With age, it would appear that the bulk of LDL cholesterol becomes small particle.

Reducing the LDL cholesterol menace to basement membranes, thereby thwarting a major risk factor to chronic inflammation, is where statins, niacin, ezetimibe, and the PCSK9 inhibitors intervene. When chronic inflammation in the interstitial space is decreased by lowering LDL cholesterol, a slew of anti-inflammatory benefits accrue. These cascading benefits intervene no matter how advanced anti-organ venues have fd. Because they can affect multiple anti-organ venues statins specifically are known to have *pleotropic anti-inflammatory effects*. This means that with enough LDL cholesterol lowering, capillary cells dance, interstitials pace sanitation improves and there is potential reversal to thrombosis, cancer genesis, recurrent infectious uprisings, autoimmune diseases and even dissipation of some end organ scarring. The pleotropic benefit works even better when anti-inflammatory lifestyle is also aligned in the process. It's amazing what exercise, seven hours of sleep, stress reduction, addiction control and treatment of elevated blood sugars and blood pressure adds to the pleotropic equation.

Any reasonable skeptic could laugh at this "too good to be true" overreach as there are just too many gaps in knowledge as to how it works. Besides, clinical studies go back and forth of whether the pleotropic actually has merit. The problem with many of these studies is that they are not properly controlled for other chronic inflammatory risks. For example, if you are studying a reduction in Parkinson Disease with statins usage and you don't also control for smoking or other addictions, blood sugar management, exercise, sleep deprivation or stress, the results will be flawed or skewed against a statin pleotropic effect.

Statins, which are the cornerstone treatment for elevated LDL cholesterol, are derived from the centuries-old Chinese medicine red rice yeast. They lower blood LDL cholesterol levels by blocking LDL cholesterol production in the liver, and are also known as *HMG-CoA reductase inhibitors*. The current list of commonly prescribed statins include rosuvastatin (Crestor), atorvastatin (Lipitor), pravastatin (Pravachol), simvastatin (Zocor), and lovastatin (Mevacor), but there are others. Reducing LDL cholesterol production lowers their blood levels thereby making fewer of them available to attach to basement membranes in the interstitial space. This enables a better chance of getting rid of them when they do arrive thereby snuffing out the risk they would cause for pluming of additional immune arsenal and the subsequent chronic interstitial space inflammation that would follow. This enables endothelial and capillary cells to retool a downshift in outer membrane fluxing of permeability, with the subsequent adjustment in mitochondrial combustion to nitric oxide following.

As interstitial space sanitation improves and the immune arsenal once again becomes purposed to capillary cell choreography instead of an anti-organ venue, the anti-inflammatory pleotropic effects occur. This is of course if other anti-inflammatory lifestyles are also note being ignored.

Whereas statins block LDL cholesterol production in the liver, niacin blocks LDL production in both liver and fat cells by affecting a different set of enzymes. Ezetimibe (Zetia) lowers blood plasma LDL cholesterol by blocking its absorption through the intestinal epithelial cells. By *blocking glucose (sugar) utilization* in LDL cholesterol production, niacin and statins can bias increases in blood sugars, thereby biasing an increased risk towards diabetes. This makes lifestyle interventions regarding diet and exercise mandatory when taking stains or niacin. PCSK9 inhibitors lower blood LDL cholesterol levels by inducing LDL cholesterol transport back into the liver cells for catabolic breakdown. When appropriate, adding ezetimibe or a PCSK9 inhibitor to a statin to further reduce elevated LDL cholesterol levels confers additional anti-inflammatory benefit, which likely translates to even better disease treatment outcomes involving anti-organ venues.

For more than fifty years, *niacin,* or vitamin B$_3$, has been used to lower blood LDL (or "bad") cholesterol, increase HDL (or "good" anti-inflammatory cholesterol), lower lipo(a) (also known as lipoprotein (a), a sticky proinflammatory free radical fat), and lower serum triglycerides (yet another proinflammatory free radical blood plasma fat). While niacin moves all of the cholesterol sub particles in the right anti-inflammatory direction this does not translate to improved benefits that would occur from just lowering LDL cholesterol. Since niacin lowering of LDL cholesterol is not as potent as statin lowering, it can't be considered a first line preferred intervention. Because of its superiority as an anti-inflammatory niacin should be used only in niche situations, such as when there are significant elevations in lipo(a) coupled with a strong family history of premature heart attacks and death. In this setting, it can be assumed that elevated lipo(a) is dangerous and very proinflammatory. Since niacin is the only currently available means of lowering lipo(a) it should be deployed at maximum doses of 2-3 grams daily to aggressively bring lipo(a) levels down.

Ezetimibe is a relative newcomer in the expanding repertoire of LDL cholesterol–reduction treatments. It lowers LDL cholesterol about 20–30 percent, which is similar to what the older statins and niacin can accomplish. Unlike niacin, when additional LDL cholesterol lowering is required, ezetimibe can be combined with a statin to confer additional anti-inflammatory benefit.

PCSK9 inhibitors are the newcomer to the LDL cholesterol–lowering group. As they are very expensive with the clinical kinks still being worked out, it would appear they have efficacy in situations where LDL cholesterol lowering is stubborn or can't be achieved with combinations of statins or ezetimibe. They require a once or twice a month injection as it is expected that using PCSK9 inhibitors will confer anti-inflammatory benefits to LDL cholesterol lowering in a small group of patients that previously could not get to LDL cholesterol lowering goal.

While there is considerable buzz in using statins for their anti-inflammatory pleotropic effects, a cousin to niacin, *nicotinamide,* when coupled with ingested vitamin D, can substantially reduce skin cancer incidence. This Australian study showed reductions in all types of skin cancer including melanoma. It would suggest that niacin's cousin coupled with vitamin D can induce pleotropic effects.

Higher doses of the more potent statins, atorvastatin and rosuvastatin, further reduce *angina pectoris* (heart pain) and prevent death from heart attacks and strokes, presumably by a more rigorous reduction in LDL cholesterol levels compared to other statins in those with serious preexisting large vessel obstructive plaque. They also stabilize patency and improve success of vascular interventions involving the placement of stents or bypass grafts. Other studies link higher doses of statins to reduced incidence of atrial fibrillation. Still others are linking statins to benefits in cancer treatment, reducing exacerbations of COPD and asthma, as well as reducing stroke and dementia incidence risks.

Side effects of treatment with statins or niacin are linked directly to low CoQ10 levels. This is because statins, and to some extent niacin, block CoQ10 production. As Co Q10 levels decrease, mitochondria become less efficient in making energy. This affects skeletal muscle by causing muscle pain and weakness. In rare cases, skeletal muscle can actually break down to cause *rhabdomyolysis,* which does not bode well for kidney function. When this occurs, the statin should be discontinued, and if necessary intravenous fluid resuscitation and even dialysis maybe required to restore kidney function.

In those with fatty liver, cirrhosis, and chronic hepatitis C or B infections, ezetimibe may be a better choice to lower LDL cholesterol.

Some if not all of the skeletal muscle side effects can be prevented by supplementing with CoQ10, lowering the dose of statin, or changing to an entirely different statin. Drinking even modest amounts of alcohol should be discouraged when taking statins as they can increase liver inflammation and potentiate muscle weakness.

Summary

There is no excuse for not addressing the chronic end-organ interstitial-space inflammation that is menaced by elevated LDL blood plasma cholesterol. Statins are safe and very effective in reducing LDL cholesterol free radicals within the interstitial space. Doing so, allows capillary cell outer membranes to flux permeability downward enabling a return to their dance. Subsequent mitochondrial nitric oxide combustion increases rejuvenation and improved interstitial space sanitation is on its way.

Dosing of all these medicines requires clinical acumen and close attention of guidelines. Excessive LDL cholesterol lowering may carry its own set of risks and suggests that there can be too much of a good thing. Best-practice guidelines call for LDL cholesterol to be lowered to between 70–100 mg/dl, with lowering closer to the 70 range in those with diabetes, previous coronary stents or bypass grafts, recurrent angina, or very high coronary calcium scores.

Lowering blood plasma LDL cholesterol reduces chronic interstitial space and endothelial/capillary cell basement membrane inflammation, which enables endothelial and capillary cells to flux their outer membrane permeability and pendulum swing mitochondrial combustion. Resuming the capillary cell dance confers a return of a more optimal interstitial space homeostasis that nullifies anti-organ intent while also facilitating improved end organ function and rejuvenation. Doing so causes pleotropic benefits to the interstitial space involving reductions in thrombosis, cancer, infections, autoimmune complexes and even scarring. No time like the present to get the capillary cells back on the dance floor!

Aspirin and Other Platelet Inhibitors

Aspirin has been used for more than a century to relieve pain and treat fever, but in the last half century, its most important benefit has been discovered. Aspirin reduces chronic inflammation within interstitial spaces. In those with preexisting chronic inflammation and already inflamed endothelial- and capillary-cell basement membranes, 81 milligrams per day of aspirin blocks the building momentum of pro-clotting biases within the interstitial spaces and blood plasma. By blocking platelet adhesion to an already inflamed or ulcerated membrane surface prevents clotting cascades that lead to a *thrombosis* or a potential *complete occlusion* to a vessel lumen. Occlusions block blood flow and can be life threatening, as blood-flow upstream to the thrombosis is cutoff, thereby causing a sometimes dramatic reduction of oxygen and nutrient to the upstream interstitial space and end organ.

Platelets are cells made in the bone marrow, circulate in the bloodstream, and along with clotting factors produced in the liver and when activated, induce blood plasma to clot. As part of a chronic inflammatory cascade and anti-organ venue, they can be pulled (transported) from the blood plasma through zombied capillary cells and into the interstitial spaces of end organs. It is in this setting which is fueled by vascular inflammatory free-radical seeds and the expanding immune arsenal response towards them, where aspirin intervention can be beneficial, even lifesaving. By blocking platelet adherence to a chronically inflamed membrane surface, aspirin prevents the anti-organ escalation of thrombosis and perhaps the display of other end organ white flag venues.

Clotting (thrombosis) risks leading to an end organ hypoxic- ischemic event can occur in any interstitial space but are particularly worrisome to end organs that are oxygen sensitive, such as brain, heart or retina. In these vulnerable end organs, even small vessel clots induce end organ injury to cause angina, heart attack, transient ischemic attack(s) (mini stroke) or macular degeneration. Over time, these "mini attacks" aggregate their effect leading to substantial end organ compromise that include heart failure, dementia and blindness. Taking a baby aspirin (81 mg) daily, beginning at age fifty, can predictably reduce the incidence of all sorts of vascular occlusive events, including heart attacks and strokes, by upwards of 30 percent over extended periods of time.

What taking aspirin for a period of 5 or more years, anti-inflammatory pleotropic benefits occur, suggesting sustained benefits against different anti-organ venues. Taking a daily baby aspirin appears to reduce and even assist in treatment to cancers of the colon, breast, and prostate with the list expanding. Like statins, metformin and beta blockers, aspirin has become *add- on* in some chemotherapy regimens for treating cancer.

But why should aspirin use start at age 50? It is because at age 50 chronic inflammation has established a beach head in the interstitial spaces and basement membranes throughout the arterial tree. Imaging shows the beginning of basement membrane thickening in larger vessels as well as early calcium buildup in heart valves, all of which increase clotting risk and thrombosis. This risk further escalates as addictions come to a head, weight is gained, exercise vanishes, sleep deprivation increases and stress advances. All of these issues converge in most adult at age 50. When they do aspirin, and other platelet inhibitors, such as *ticagrelor* and *clopidogrel,* can substantially reduce thrombotic risk. The benefits to aspirin and other blood thinners actually increase with age as long as they don't cause excessive bleeding. The risk of bleeding becomes the number one contraindication to use aspirin or other blood thinners.

While aspirin's anti-thrombotic benefits are coupled with other anti-inflammatory behaviors and treatments, their benefits increase by another rung. For example, when daily aspirin use is coupled with a statin to lower LDL cholesterol, tobacco and drug abstinence, exercise, and a Mediterranean diet, thrombotic events and cancer incidence decrease even further. Over time this translates to fewer strokes and heart attacks and their frightful outcomes of heart failure, dementia and macular blindness. It also means additional pleotropic benefits that include reductions in the incidence of several cancers, and serious systemic infections requiring hospitalization for treatment. (View graphs

1-5, appendix). All of this implies that even when vascular inflammatory seeds have created enough chronic inflammation to torture the interstitial space and advance anti-organ venues, anti-inflammatory intervention can cause dramatic reversals of fortune. Even wellness can make a difference when the anti-organ cat is out of the bag. As long as capillary cells can get back on the dance floor to pivot and swing, there is a chance that interstitial space inflammatory chaos can be reversed. Reversing chronic inflammation is another way of saying capillary and endothelial cell rejuvenation which translates to anti-aging.

On a molecular level, aspirin blocks platelet activation to cause adhesion by blocking prostaglandin production within platelets of *thromboxane A2*. Biases to increased platelet production of thromboxane A2 occurs with chronic interstitial space inflammation. Without thromboxane A2, platelets don't adhere and completion of a clotting cascade to thrombosis does not occur.

Daily low dose 81 mg aspirin is usually taken with food because of the risk of stomach bleeding. Bleeding issues get complex when aspirin is coupled other prescription blood thinners or with over the counter fish oils or ginkgo biloba. Too much blood thinning and bleeding risk escalates. Don't hide supplement usage with your health care provider. Substantial bruising of the skin without verifiable trauma is a sign that there may be too much blood thinning.

Summary

Aspirin therapy (daily dose of 81 mg) is an essential add-on treatment to limit pro clotting biases and subsequent thrombosis and hypoxic-ischemic events linked to chronic interstitial space inflammation. When utilized with other anti-inflammatory treatments, they provide strong impetus for endothelial and capillary-cell outer-membranes to resume permeability pivoting and dance their two-step with mitochondria to swing combustion to nitric oxide. Doing so, begins a renewal of endothelial and capillary cell infrastructure thereby setting the stage for their rejuvenation. Anti-inflammatory momentum builds to suppress anti-organ venues as order is restored in the interstitial space. The blocking of platelet adherence become even more valuable when incorporated into a team anti-inflammatory approach involving lifestyle, other medicines and supplements.

ACEs/ARBs and Selected Antihypertensives

Like aspirin and statins, *ACEs* (*angiotensin converting enzyme inhibitors*) and *ARBs* (*angiotensin receptor blockers*), also block the ravages of chronic interstitial space inflammation to aid and abet the capillary cell dance. In this case it involves shear caused from higher blood pressures within the lumens of blood vessels. Higher blood pressures cause increases in *shear stress, which perpetuates friction induced membrane injury.* Adding an ACE or ARB treatment lowers blood pressure by blocking the effects of a potent vasoconstrictor, *angiotensin II.* Blocking angiotensin II, reduces shear friction by decreasing intraluminal pressures in larger arteries and arterioles. This is induced by the relaxing of smooth muscle cells that surround the endothelial cells of large vessel lumens. As they relax, vessel lumens dilate and blood pressure within them decreases. As pressure decreases, *shear-friction stress* and the injury it causes to endothelial cell outer membranes cells is reduced.

Increased shear stress can be both a cause and effect of hypertension (also known as high blood pressure). Increased shear perpetuates endothelial- and capillary-cell outer membrane injury by creating a chronic immune arsenal response towards the injured membrane surface. As the inflammatory plume expands, it increases interstitial space inflammation and disrupts the endothelial cell's relationship to the adjoining smooth muscle cells. The mechanics of this disruption, through the expansion of the immune arsenal plum, is similar to how other vascular inflammatory free radicals incite chronic interstitial space inflammation. Thus shear stress becomes its own free radical and is birthed by the seeding of other vascular inflammatory free radicals. In other words, tobacco toxins, AGEs, LDL cholesterol, and lipo(a), among other free radicals, further contribute to increased shear. As such, hypertension from shear injury, with the subsequent increase in angiotensin II in the bloodstream, becomes a manifestation of accumulating vascular inflammatory free radicals within interstitial spaces of the arterial tree.

Angiotensin II is a potent *vasoconstrictor* that increases in the blood as a result of chronic interstitial space inflammation. Liver, kidney and lung end organs work together to regulate the expansion or contraction of angiotensin II activation based on signals from arterial endothelium. With chronic interstitial space inflammation the endothelium are duped to misread blood flow dynamics. Instead of messaging a reduction they instead send messages to the liver, lung and kidney to increase activation of angiotensin II. Once activated, it causes smooth muscle cells to contract around endothelium causing profound increases in intraluminal pressures and subsequent endothelial cell outer membrane injury. The injury doubles down on further interstitial space inflammation which enables the coalescing chronic inflammatory matrix to pursue pirating of the endothelial and capillary cell outer membranes. From here the events become predictable. There is a diffuse endothelial and capillary cell fail, as aggregate vascular inflammatory risks and the hypertension they have affected or caused, become the fuel to the anti-organ elephant in the room.

ACEs and ARBs decrease the mismanaged angiotensin II by either blocking its *production* (ACEs) or blocking its *targeted effect* (ARBs). In the case of endothelial cells it blocks angiotensin induced smooth-muscle cell contraction which allows arterial lumens to once again expand thereby lowering blood pressure. Lowering shear injury and blood pressure by blocking the effects of angiotensin II can be even more effective when other chronic inflammatory free radicals such as LDL cholesterol, AGEs or tobacco toxins are also reduced. In other words without an all-out assault on vascular inflammatory free radicals, blood pressures will still be biased to increase from ongoing and progressive interstitial space inflammation.

When blood pressures normalizes (less than or equal to 140/85), the implication is that shear injury no longer is adding to the chronic inflammatory woes of the interstitial spaces of the arterial tree. For this effect to be truly beneficial long term, other vascular inflammatory free radicals must also be reduced. Any chronic inflammatory activity within interstitial space that blocks the smooth muscle-endothelial cell relationship will contribute to hypertension and increased shear injury.

Other medications that lower blood pressure and reduce shear stress can produce similar shear reductions to endothelial and capillary cell outer membranes. Well known antihypertensives, such as *beta-blockers* or *calcium channel blockers,* as their name imply, can reduce shear stress from different mechanisms other than blocking angiotensin II.

Blocking angiotensin II over time can have pleotropic effects on the interstitial spaces of end organs. When coupled with exercise, aspirin, statins, tobacco withdrawal and a Mediterranean diet, ACEs or ARBS potentiate reductions in anti-organ venues that include end organ interstitial space scarring and thrombosis and reduced hypoxic-ischemic events. Since reducing shear injury is so dependent on reducing other vascular inflammatory free radicals, other pleotropic benefits from lowering blood pressure with antihypertensives alone is hard to prove.

Recent guidelines on treating hypertension are changing, reflecting a more aggressive approach in preventing the consequences of persistently higher blood pressures. Even modest elevations in blood pressure, which in the past were thought to be normal, are now recognized as inducing shear injury. On the other hand, overzealous treatment of high blood pressure must be moderated, particularly in the elderly, when fall risk increases as blood pressures fall upon assuming an upright posture. When it comes to blood pressure management, a fine line must be drawn as to what is best for a given patient with ideal blood pressures scaled to individual patient risks.

In addition to controlling blood pressure with anti-hypertensives, even better control is facilitated with regular exercise, weight control (BMI index less than 30), stress reduction, treatment of sleep disorders, reduced salt intake, improving hemoglobin A1C levels, reduced LDL cholesterol, and tobacco, alcohol and drug abstinence. Elevations in blood pressure are often an early clinical cue that one or more of vascular inflammatory free radicals are producing enough endothelial and capillary cell membrane inflammation to increase blood pressure. Addressing blood pressure elevations earlier in life, and particularly with reference to reducing circulating vascular inflammatory free radicals, will postpone end-organ complications down the road.

As with all blood pressure medications, once ACE and ARB treatment has been initiated, careful dose titration is required to optimize blood pressure control without side effects. Measurements of blood electrolytes, blood sugars, serum lipids, and kidney and liver function should be performed periodically. Side effects of ACE and ARB medicines include cough (worse with ACE inhibitors) and rarely a serious swelling of the face and body (*angioedema*). Angioedema can be serious as it could lead to throat obstruction and asphyxiation. Urgent withdrawal from the medicine and occasional airway management is required. If a dry, hacking cough occurs, and is not due to an infection or allergy, switching from an ACE to an ARB should eliminate the cough.

Summary

When blood pressure is elevated, angiotensin II is likely an active participant. Blocking angiotensin II, by and ACE or ARB, lowers blood pressure and reliably reverses shear stress–induced endothelial and capillary cell injury. When coupled with reductions in other vascular inflammatory free radicals, a potent recipe evolves to encourage the reintroduction of the endothelial and capillary cell dance, the blocking of chronic interstitial space inflammation and the venues of the anti-organ. As might be expected, reducing high blood pressure and the shear stress that it causes by blocking angiotensin II decreases the frequency of strokes and heart attacks and the outcomes which include heart failure and dementia. Other pleotropic benefits occur when coupled with reductions of other vascular inflammatory free radicals.

Metformin

Metformin, which is derived from a French lilac (goat's-rue), has been used in Europe over the last 50 years to lower blood sugars in the treatment of adult diabetes. It received FDA approval for use in the United States sometime after that. Metformin reduces chronic inflammation within interstitial spaces by *blocking gluconeogenesis* in all cells but with major metabolic impact coming from doing so in the liver, intestines, and kidney. Blocking the conversion of pyruvate to glucose by gluconeogenesis shifts energy substrate utilized by mitochondria towards pyruvate and hence sugar utilization. This reduces insulin resistance and blood sugars. Since metformin also reduces apatite and hence calories ingested, it has a double whammy effect to lowering blood sugars. The net effect is to increase pyruvate mitochondrial combustion, reduce calories ingested, while also decreasing circulating free-radical *AGEs* (advanced glycation end products).

Decreasing AGEs reduces endothelial and capillary cell outer membrane inflammation by limiting the likelihood of its attachment and subsequent silencing it causes of receptor function and the pluming of immune arsenal towards it. By increasing pyruvate over fatty acid combustion in mitochondria, there is less production of superoxide free radical exhaust. This means there is less risk of mitochondrial DNA superoxide cross- linkage, which bodes well long term for mitochondrial survival. By reducing calories ingested, some of the risk of fatty acid buildup within cells is reduced.

By blocking gluconeogenesis, metformin induces a similar metabolic fate within cells that mimics exercise or *low-calorie diets*. One key to metformin induced less glucose production and more pyruvate utilization by mitochondria is what happens to fatty acids. As fatty acids accumulate, beta oxidation within mitochondria gets blocked forcing fatty acids into different directions and purposes within the cell. This could include synthesis of lipoproteins or incorporation into membrane surfaces. By reducing multiple vascular inflammatory free radical risks, this derivative of the French lilac, becomes a pluripotent antagonist to chronic inflammation.

Because of this it would be expected that metformin has anti-inflammatory pleotropic benefits. It reduces thrombotic events (strokes, TIAs, angina pectoris, heart attack), has produced favorable effects in the prevention and treatment of polycystic ovaries, and has been used as an add on in the treatment of several cancers. Preliminary investigation suggests benefit in blocking progression of dementia. It may have favorable benefits as add -on in treating certain autoimmune diseases. It decreases fatty liver, improves kidney filtering, and can decrease macular degeneration of the retina. Metformin also improves lung alveolar gas exchange and has shown benefit to reduce adverse outcomes linked to asthma and COPD. Even the mobilization of bacteria in the blood stream, also known as sepsis, is decreased with metformin. Metformin's pleotropic anti-inflammatory effects cascade against chronic inflammatory venues in ways that are not expected but welcomed.

Although metformin is currently FDA approved for treatment of type 2 adult-onset diabetes, it is being used "off label" (or in investigation protocols) as adjuvant therapy for a variety of other serious inflammatory and medical conditions involving the treatment and prevention of scarring, thrombosis, cancer, infections and autoimmune disorders. Metformin cannot be used as a supplement, but is often prescribed in low doses in prediabetes (hemoglobin A1C 5.7-6.4) where chronic inflammation is still occurring.

Metformin must be prescribed carefully, as it can cause hypoglycemia and occasionally increase risk for *lactic acidosis*. Lactic acidosis can be serious as it can affect blood electrolytes and PH to sequentially disrupt heart rhythms and increase respirations. When lactic acidosis occurs, metformin should be immediately withdrawn. Lactic acidosis can increase when imaging studies utilize contrast dyes or when there is preexisting kidney damage. Caution with metformin use is advised with either of these situations. Metformin has been associated with B12 deficiency and this B vitamin may need supplementing. Alcohol use, when taking metformin should be discouraged, as the two of them used together could potentiate liver toxicity.

Summary

By blocking glucose production from pyruvate in a process known as gluconeogenesis, metformin has become a cornerstone treatment for adult-onset diabetes. Its benefits cascade to decrease multiple vascular inflammatory free radicals that contribute to absolute reductions in chronic interstitial space inflammation. In this manner, metformin ushers the return of endothelia and capillary cell dance, which then facilitates the return of capillary cell homeostasis, interstitial space sanitation and end organ performance. All this occurs while pushing back on anti-organ venues. In this manner, metformin becomes part of a rejuvenating antidote to chronic illnesses, fatigue, pain and aging.

Nitrates, Arginine, and Citrulline

A major theme in *Rejuvenation* is that chronic interstitial space inflammation is the cause of interstitial space decay and the subsequent development of illness, fatigue, pain and aging. Chronic inflammation takes advantage through the persistent occupation of the interstitial space by vascular inflammatory free radicals. As the stew brews, it coalesces to form an inflammatory matrix to take ownership of the interstitial space by capturing the interest of the immune arsenal and mesenchymal cells. With increasing inflammatory momentum, the inflammatory matrix uses different pieces of the immune arsenal to pirate the capillary cell outer membranes to take full control of the interstitial space. This enables the anti-organ to begin initiating different disease processes, through a series of different preselected venues, based on inherent end organ vulnerabilities and genetic profiles. As the diseases mount, the anti-organ becomes increasingly more powerful as it uses more immune arsenal to his advantage. As this is occurring, the end organ is shrinking.

Except for is use of oxygen, mitochondrial nitric oxide combustion (see appendix, figure 17) requires a completely different set of precursors, substrates and enzymes, as compared to energy combustion. It also creates a different free radical exhaust making the two combustion cycles completely different. This enables clear feedback loop message to on –off switches involving membranes and other organelles, as the mechanics of the two different types of mitochondrial combustion are entirely different.

When endothelia and capillary cell mitochondria shift to nitric oxide combustion, it utilizes the amino acids *arginine* and *citrulline*, a hydrogen carrier (NADP-nicotinamide adenine dinucleotide phosphate), cofactors such as vitamin D, oxygen and the enzyme *nitric oxide synthetase*. Nitric oxide production *does not* involve the cytochromes of the inner membrane or the Krebs cycle and it does not produce superoxide exhaust. Instead, activated nitric oxide synthetase *blocks* cytochrome electron movement to shut down energy combustion. This forms the basis for the pendulum swing of combustion, which responds to outer membranes shifts in energy demands based on fluxing permeability to immune arsenal.

The back and forth mitochondrial combustion of energy and nitric oxide forms the basis for interstitial space hygiene, capillary and end organ cell renewal, as well as disease prevention (wellness), reduction in fatigue and pain and antiaging.

Besides reducing inflammatory free radical burden within the interstitial space, an alternative way to goose deficient capillary cell nitric oxide production is to "push" it by *flooding their mitochondria* with nitric oxide precursors. This would include ingesting large amounts of arginine, citrulline, and nitrates. Goosing nitric oxide production *temporizes* mitochondrial pendulum swinging but does not address the interstitial space free radical burden. Unless free radicals are also reduced, nitric oxide pushing will eventually fail. Therefore, pushing nitric oxide production should be viewed as a *bridge* that facilitates a more robust nitric oxide production when vascular free radical volumes are also being reduced in the interstitial space.

Whereas ingesting *citrulline* and *arginine* requires activated nitric oxide synthetase to produce nitric oxide, *nitrate* and *nitroglycerin* ingestion can bypass nitric oxide synthetase by utilizing the enzyme *aldehyde dehydrogenase*. This enzyme converts these substrates to nitric oxide without requiring nitric oxide synthetase activation. This means that nitric oxide can be produced through this pathway when capillary cell mitochondria are busy combusting energy. This alternative pathway becomes critically important in settings where end organs, such as heart muscle, scream for more oxygen while capillary cell mitochondria are preoccupied combusting energy.

This would commonly occur in hypoxic- ischemic events (angina) where heart muscle cell interstitial space is inflamed from lack of oxygen, capillary cell outer membranes are in permeability free fall, and their mitochondria are cranking energy to support the persistent push of permeability. In this crisis situation, involving a severely compromised heart muscle cell, ingesting a rapidly absorbable nitrate or nitroglycerin will use the alternative pathway and be converted to nitric oxide in capillary cell mitochondria. Ingesting nitrates therefore becomes an important treatment of acute of chronic lack of end organ oxygen supply, but does not reframe the vascular free radicals causes that have produced the crisis. Whereas nitrates address crisis management, citrulline or arginine are better utilized in boosting nitric oxide production when inflammatory free radical populations are simultaneously being reduced.

Summary

For arginine or citrulline supplementation to be effective, other lifestyle adjustments should have already been initiated to efforts to jump start the capillary cell dance, flux permeability and swing mitochondrial combustion to nitric oxide. Using these precursors in this setting should produce a more robust nitric oxide response that could cause a more rapid repletion of mitochondrial volumes and outer membrane receptors. This could help even in compromised situations where chronic inflammation had caused a significant reduction in capillary cell mitochondrial volumes. Oral nitrates utilize a different nitric oxide production pathway which makes them effective in emergent or crisis situations where end organ cells need oxygen fast or they risk dying.

Do nitrates have pleotropic benefits against anti-organ venues? Probably. Ingesting nitrates, when coupled with other anti-inflammatory interventions, not only improves outcomes involving all kinds of heart and brain conditions related to chronic lack of oxygen, but also has benefits in fighting cancer. Adding nitrates, to other standard prostate cancer treatments, confers additional benefit in reducing prostate cancer progression. This may just be the beginning to nitrate interventions in disease treatment or prevention.

Nitrates have FDA-approved indications to treat and prevent angina pectoris (heart pain) and are also approved for treatment of hypertension and heart failure. Different nitrates are being used off label in the treatment of other medical conditions. Arginine (or L-arginine) and citrulline are considered supplements, and as expected, currently have no FDA-approved indications for disease treatment or prevention.

Nitrate side effects include flushing, dizziness, and headaches. When nitrates are used regularly, these annoying side effects tend to diminish. Switching to a longer-acting nitrate or decreasing the dose often reduces side effects.

Supplementing arginine/ citrulline into the mitochondrial apparatus, when vascular inflammatory free radicals are being reduced, could fast-track more comprehensive capillary cell rejuvenation. Doing so could enable the capillary cell to better reestablish itself in pacing interstitial space sanitation while re- expanding end organ function.

Vitamins D and K$_2$

Up until about 20 years ago, *vitamin D* was thought to be primarily involved in bone health in the treatment and prevention of soft bones, also known as *osteoporosis*. In the last twenty years, that has changed dramatically. Vitamin D is now known to be a cofactor to multiple on-off switches, and feedback loop mechanics involving the outer membranes, mitochondria, nucleus and other organelles.

In humans, active vitamin D requires adequate absorption of vitamin D precursors through the intestines, an ultraviolet light conversion through the skin, and one additional molecular addition through the kidney. Deficiency in one or more stages of this triangle accounts for vitamin D deficiency states in up to 75 percent of older adults.

Vitamin D works on both sides of mitochondrial combustion, but perhaps the most important function is serving as a *cofactor* for activation of nitric oxide synthetase. By facilitating nitric oxide synthetase activation, vitamin D deficiency becomes a *rate-limiting* component to facilitating a robust nitric oxide production. Since capillary cell nitric oxide production is already biased downward from chronic inflammation in the elderly, vitamin D deficiency further compounds its reduction.

By extension, when nitric oxide is being combusted, reduced vitamin D levels blunt rejuvenation of endothelial and capillary cells. This ultimately translates to a less complete sanitation of the interstitial space and rejuvenation of the end organ. Vitamin D therefore becomes the rejuvenating vitamin, a pivotal cofactor to nitric oxide combustion and subsequent rejuvenation of capillary-cells and their partners.

It is postulated that as vitamin D levels fall, nitric oxide synthetase activity, which is already compromised, decreases even further. As chronic interstitial space inflammation preoccupies the interstitial space, capillary cell outer membrane permeability and mitochondrial energy combustion, not only is nitric oxide production decreased, but with vitamin D deficiency, it decreases even further. This bodes poorly for the future of the interstitial space and the end organ. Cascades of different interstitial space diseases expand like wild fire.

Recently, another vitamin known as *vitamin K_2,* has been shown to assist vitamin D in some of its cofactor functions, specifically related to calcium shuttling. By facilitating the shuttling of calcium away from endothelial and capillary cell basement membranes surfaces, vitamin K_2 helps prevent calcium from precipitating into chronic inflammatory plumes on membrane surfaces. Instead, calcium remobilizes elsewhere, either back into cells to be stored or transported and attached to bony matrix. By facilitating calcium mobilization away from already inflamed outer membranes, vitamin K2 becomes a key anti-inflammatory participant. The combination of vitamin D3 and vitamin K2 have become attractive supplements to improving bone turgor.

Vitamin K2 is part of a family of vitamin K vitamins that have different functions but which can cross react with one another. For this reason, these vitamins must be used with caution when complex medical conditions require different vitamin Ks to be blocked or augmented.

As with many vitamins and antioxidants, vitamins D and K_2 blood levels usually decrease with age and therefore merit supplementation. In the case of vitamin D, blood levels should be checked periodically and the vitamin dose adjusted based on its deficiency. With vitamin K2, dosing is more empiric and must be performed with an understanding of how other forms of vitamin K are being treated. For example giving Vitamin K2 could cross react to block warfarin's effect on vitamin K1, thereby nullifying an important blood thinning effect. Similarly, taking vitamin D could be dangerous when calcium levels are already elevated in the blood from different kinds of cancer or parathyroid hormone elevations. The use of these supplements should therefore not be random but carefully calculated into a specific therapeutic regime.

Currently, there are no FDA-approved indications for taking vitamin K_2. Vitamin D_3 is FDA approved to treat vitamin D deficiency. If there are no clinical contraindications, vitamins D and K_2 could be taken together for their synergistic effects on improving the efficiency of nitric oxide combustion and calcium ion shuttling.

Does vitamin D have pleotropic benefits to anti-organ venues? Based on how it integrates into cellular metabolism to improve homeostasis, one would think so. Studies are now demonstrating a relationship between vitamin D supplementation and the reduced incidence of certain cancers. Other reports have linked supplementation of vitamins D and K_2 either separate or together, to reductions in depression, dementia, sepsis, heart failure, heart arrhythmias, falls and hip fractures. Vitamin D supplementation has been linked to fewer hospital admissions (or readmissions) for treatment of serious infections (sepsis) or syncopal events (sudden loss of consciousness). The inference suggests that these supplements help to reduce chronic inflammatory interstitial space reach, revitalize the capillary cell dance, stoke combustion of nitric oxide, and rejuvenate capillary and endothelial cells and their partners. All of this while reducing anti-organ venues.

Summary

Vitamin D, by facilitating mitochondrial nitric oxide synthetase activation and a more robust nitric oxide production, supports a more complete capillary- and endothelial-cell rejuvenation. It becomes even more effective when chronic inflammation within interstitial spaces is also being simultaneously tamed. Adding vitamin K_2 to vitamin D doubles down on the anti-inflammatory benefit by shuttling calcium away from endothelia and capillary cell membranes thereby biasing decreases in membrane permeability while reducing the risk for calcium deposition on interstitial-space basement membranes. Resetting a more-robust capillary cell nitric oxide production becomes a key piece to its reemergence as a facilitator of interstitial space hygiene. This enables potential cascades of remission from anti-organ venues, fatigue and pain.

Coenzyme Q$_{10}$ (Ubiquinone)

Coenzyme Q_{10} (CoQ_{10}) has a *dual function* in the mitochondria of capillary, endothelial, and end-organ cells. It *facilitates electron transport,* leading to more efficient combustion of energy, while also acting as an *antioxidant* to remove toxic free radical exhaust from within the mitochondrial matrix. This dual function of facilitating electron transfer to increase energy production efficiency, while also protecting the mitochondrial DNA from free radical exhaust damage, makes CoQ_{10} indispensable. Unfortunately, with advanced age, chronic inflammation, anti-organ venues, and use of statin medications, CoQ_{10} levels can decrease precipitously in all cells. In these settings, supplementing CoQ_{10} is mandatory.

In figure 2 in the appendix, *ubiquinone* (also known as UQ or CoQ_{10}), plays a critical role in electron transfer through the cytochrome system (I–III) within the mitochondrial inner membrane. CoQ_{10} is required in all end-organ cells for energy combustion, but particularly in those that must combust large amounts of energy to support increases in function, such as brain, heart, retina and skeletal muscle.

When capillary cell mitochondria swing combustion to nitric oxide,

CoQ_{10} becomes an antioxidant to help clean up superoxide and other free radicals produced form energy combustion. By doing so, it helps prevent *free radical chain reactions*. This means that ubiquinone is busy, no matter what the mitochondria are combusting. When energy is in high demand, CoQ10 transfers electrons. When nitric oxide synthesis increases, it neutralizes free radicals. In this sense it serves as an energy facilitator and free radical buffer.

Ubiquinone teams up with other antioxidants—glutathione, vitamins C and E, alpha-lipoic acid (ALA), and manganese superoxide dismutase (MnSOD), among others—to prevent free-radical chain reactions. Free radical chain reactions occur when a free radical transfers a charge to a neutral molecule to make a charged free radical molecule. The free radical created in the chain, can cause its own set of damages to different membrane surfaces. Thus free radical chain reactions act as a carpet bomb to capillary cell infrastructure and membrane surfaces. Utilizing a *team* of antioxidants to block free radical chain reactions prevents carpet bombing. Since CoQ_{10} can penetrate both fat- and water-soluble membranes, it becomes a flexible antioxidant team player to neutralize free radicals in many locations.

In those where deficiency is likely, ubiquinone should be supplemented. Doing so, increases the efficiency of energy production while reducing clustered free radical intracellular damage. It works best when vascular inflammatory free radical burden is also being reduced.

CoQ_{10} being a supplement is not FDA approved for disease treatment or prevention. In the right clinical setting, supplementing at doses of 200 milligrams or more per day can go a long way to improving endothelial, capillary and end organ cell performance. There are very few side effects or known drug interactions with CoQ_{10} supplementing. As with most supplements, it should be used with caution in those being treated for cancer and should not be used in adolescents, children, or pregnant women.

Summary

CoQ$_{10,}$ when coupled with lifestyle and other treatments to reduce the effects of chronic inflammation, becomes powerful support to capillary and endothelial cell homoeostasis. When statins are being used, to prevent muscle fatigue or pain, it should be an automatic add-on.

Sirtuin Activators

The supplements *resveratrol, pterostilbene,* and *nicotinamide riboside* (NR) have beneficial effects on capillary cell mitochondria by activating *selective sirtuins.* Sirtuins, like viamin D, can facilitate activation of nitric oxide synthetase to foster a more robust production of nitric oxide. As such, sirtuins 1 and 3 are switched on when capillary cell outer membranes down shift permeability to inflammatory mediators, as a result of reduced interstitial space vascular inflammatory free radical burden. as a result of reduced interstitial space inflammatory momentum. Like vitamin D, by facilitating nitric oxide synthetase, certain sirtuins can cause a more robust nitric oxide production leading to a more comprehensive rejuvenation of the capillary cell, and by extension, its partners.

The sirtuin on switch to induce nitric oxide synthetase activity becomes less active with advanced age and chronic interstitial space inflammation. When the mitochondrial combustion swing does occur, it can be short lived and puny, substantially cutting into nitric oxide production and subsequent benefit. Therefore, supplementing sirtuin activators may induce a more robust nitric oxide response if vascular free radical momentum is also being addressed. The combination of a reduced interstitial space free radical burden with more robust nitric oxide combustion, births the likelihood of an improved rejuvenation and a faster more comprehensive return of capillary cell dancing and homeostasis. Interstitial space sanitation and end organ vitality return as anti- organ venues recede.

Whereas resveratrol and pterostilbene are found naturally in grapes and berries, nicotinamide riboside (NR) is found in high concentrations in cow's milk. NR is part of the vitamin B_3 (niacin) vitamin family. In addition to activating sirtuins, NR is a precursor to the production of mitochondrial hydrogen transporters - NAD (*nicotinamide adenine dinucleotide*) and NADP (*nicotinamide adenine dinucleotide phosphate*). In this sense, NR facilitates both endpoints of mitochondrial combustion.

In addition to activating nitric oxide synthetase, sirtuin 1 and 3 activators also facilitate mitochondrial production of acetyl CoA from pyruvate and fatty acids. Acetyl CoA becomes the hub of purpose for both mitochondrial energy production and nitric oxide induction of protein synthesis for repair and replacement. When facilitating acetyl CoA production, sirtuin activators benefit capillary cell mitochondria no matter which way their combustion swings.

Sirtuin activation can also increase activity of critically important antioxidants in the mitochondrial matrix, such as *MnSOD (or SOD)*. Along with glutathione, they neutralize superoxide. In this manner, sirtuin activators increase effectiveness of nitric oxide combustion, facilitate energy combustion and protein synthesis, all while producing damage control by limiting superoxide exposures.

Consuming a daily handful of red grapes or blueberries is one way of obtaining resveratrol and pterostilbene. If these berries are not readily available or too expensive, it may be beneficial to supplement resveratrol (starting at 100 mg) and pterostilbene (starting at 10 mg). Higher doses of both, but particularly pterostilbene, can reduce insulin resistance and lower blood sugars. Nicotinamide riboside can be supplemented as well starting at doses of 250mg and then titrating to 500 milligrams per day.

Sirtuin activator dosing is almost entirely subjective and empiric. There are no FDA-approved indications to treat or prevent disease, as research is preliminary and mostly theoretical. Children, adolescents, and pregnant women should not use them. Established dosing cannot be provided, and there can be substantial variability in the quality of different supplement brands. In the big picture, it is always best to get these and other valuable nutrients from the natural world.

I believe sirtuin activators hold promise, particularly in wellness, but their often dramatic anti-aging sales pitch coupled with very preliminary and limited clinical studies demonstrating efficacy, give the appearance of an over-reach and feels gimmicky. More due diligence is recommended. Sirtuin activators can interact with prescription medicines; therefore they should be used with caution in those taking them. Any cancer diagnosis should also be a red flag, necessitating discussions about their intended use with a treating oncologist.

Summary

Activating sirtuins 1 and 3, when coupled with an anti-inflammatory lifestyle that doubles down on vascular inflammatory free radicals burdens within interstitial spaces, improves mitochondrial combustion outcomes. This cascades to include a rejuvenated capillary cell dance, which then provides momentum towards improved interstitial space sanitation and end organ function. The circle is completed when end organ and mesenchymal cells join the rejuvenating party. As anti-organ venues remit, end organ function returns, and fatigue, and pain relent.

Omega-3 Oils

Omega three oils have stirred anti-inflammatory intrigue beginning with studies decades ago on subarctic Inuit cultures. The results suggested that a diet of fatty fish reduced cardiovascular diseases or the development of inflammatory plaque in large arteries. Since then, the *omega-3 oils,* which are found in fatty salt water fish, have emerged as the basis for how these fish reduce cardiovascular mortality. When incorporated into the Mediterranean diet reductions in stroke and heart attack approach 30% from control subjects.

The omega-3 oils are composed of long fatty-acid carbon chains known primarily as *nonessential docosahexaenoic acid* (DHA) and *essential eicosapentaenoic acid* (EPA). This means EPA must be ingested, while DHA, which can be constructed in human cells from EPA. DHA is a potent multidimensional anti-inflammatory fatty acid whereas EPA benefits are limited to reducing serum triglyceride levels. Together, DHA and EPA form an anti-inflammatory dynamic duo that reduces adverse anti-organ outcomes. While these outcomes primarily involve anti-organ venues of thrombosis and hypoxic -ischemic events in oxygen sensitive end organs such as brain and heart, pleotropic benefits of fish oil are just beginning to be studied in earnest. Research trends are suggesting that fish oil from fresh fish is superior than that obtained from fish oil capsules. This would make sense due to the diversity of different capsules, the vastly different levels of EPA and DHA found in capsule form, the length of time on the shelf, and the contamination of supplements with the proinflammatory omega 6.

Omega-3 fatty acids are also known as *polyunsaturated fatty acids* (PUFAs). Besides being found at high levels in the flesh of salmon, mackerel and tuna, PUFAs are also found in in high concentrations in crustaceans, flaxseed, and nuts. With advanced age and chronic inflammation, not only do omega-3 oils decrease in the bloodstream and in all cells, but there is also less conversion of EPA to DHA.

EPA and DHA can induce anti-inflammatory momentum within interstitial spaces through several mechanisms. By lowering blood plasma triglyceride levels, they reduce inflammatory free-radical seeding into the interstitial space. By also serving as a weak blocker to platelet aggregation, PUFAs can reduce clotting bias or thrombosis risk that increases as the anti-organ begins escalating different proinflammatory venues. By incorporating into endothelial- and capillary-cell outer membranes, PUFAs can facilitate reductions in outer-membrane permeability to inflammatory mediators. By decreasing *free radical seeds, platelet adhesiveness and capillary cell outer membrane permeability to inflammatory mediators*, omega-3 fatty acids help to switch momentum away from chronic interstitial space inflammatory influences. None of these effects are like an anti-inflammatory hammer, but collectively they can help sway anti-inflammatory momentum.

In sharp contrast to omega 3 oils, omega 6 and its conversion to arachidonic acid, is a proinflammatory mediator, creates increases in capillary cell outer membrane permeability, favors clotting biases, blocks the capillary cell dance and is used by the anti-organ to support its venues. The typical western diet of highly processed fast food and sugar favors omega 6 while contracting omega three levels. As expected, as omega 6 levels increase and omega three levels decrease, anti- organ venues proliferate, end organ function declines and pain and fatigue increase concomitantly.

Omega-3 fatty acids, particularly DHA, can have other benefits. When DHA incorporates into the mitochondrial inner membrane infrastructure, it helps stabilize voltage gradients and limit unintended hydrogen ion back flow leaking into the mitochondrial matrix. Within the mitochondrial matrix, DHA can act as an antioxidant to neutralize free radicals and prevent free radical chain reactions. When DHA acts as an antioxidant, the oxidized (charged) form can attach to *peroxisome proliferator activated receptor* (PPARs). The DHA/PPAR complex then becomes a more potent free radical scavenger. By coupling with PPARs, DHA diversifies its antioxidant properties while also recycling its antioxidant benefits. By recycling its antioxidant effect through PPARs, DHA reduces its own antioxidant exhaustion, decreases free radical chain reactions, and helps to limit other antioxidant deficiencies, such as from MnSOD and glutathione.

Despite impressive anti-inflammatory range, omega-3 oils are only FDA approved to reduce elevated blood plasma triglycerides. About 10 years ago, the American Heart Association provided a strong endorsement by recommending 1–2 grams of omega three fish oil daily. They have since reduced the fervor of their endorsement as poorly controlled studies failed to show much clinical benefit in supplementing. Eating 2-3 servings per week of fatty fish on the other hand does seem to confer anti-inflammatory benefits. These discrepancies suggest that the quality control of fish oil supplement needs more scrutiny.

Side effects to fish oil supplements are dose related and include belching, nausea, and a fishy odor to breath or sweat. Reducing the dose or switching to a different brand can help eliminate side effects. Fish oil can potentially increase bleeding risk therefore it should be used with caution by those taking aspirin and/or other blood thinners. Krill oil, which contains abundant levels of omega-3, may also contain *astaxanthin,* which has its own additional antioxidant benefit. When purchasing omega three oils it is best to avoid omega six.

Summary

Because of their multifaceted anti-inflammatory and antioxidant effects, omega-3 oils facilitate reduction in chronic interstitial space inflammatory free radicals, facilitating the endothelial and capillary cell dance and frustrate anti-organ venues. Advanced age and chronic interstitial space inflammation are associated with lower blood levels of omega-3. In these settings, supplementing omega-3, or at least eating 2-3 fatty fish meals a week, should provide additional anti-inflammatory momentum. Together, when coupled with other anti-inflammatory lifestyle choices, should help jumpstart the capillary cell dance and reset a robust rejuvenation.

Magnesium

Magnesium is an essential mineral that is interwoven into the chemistry of all cells within the human body. It has an intracellular symbiotic relationship with the minerals *manganese* and *calcium,* as they can bond to similar molecules, depending on prevailing conditions. Magnesium levels can be easily measured in a blood sample and have been found to be decreased, sometimes at alarmingly low levels, in those with malnutrition, advanced age, and chronic inflammation. Magnesium levels can also increase or decrease in those with chronic kidney and liver disease, therefore it cannot be randomly supplemented.

Magnesium deficiency can be life threatening as well, particularly in conditions associated with diabetes, heart failure, heart-rhythm disturbances, and malnutrition. Deficiency in magnesium can also delay wound healing, stroke and postoperative recovery. Deficiency states can aggravate peripheral neuropathies and contribute to skeletal-muscle weakness and cramping.

Magnesium affects the functioning of capillary-cell mitochondria and their capacity to dance with outer membranes in three important ways. First, it is integral to the synthesis of both nuclear and mitochondrial DNA, as well as in stabilizing DNA infrastructure. Second, the electron transport chain and Krebs cycle utilize magnesium as a cofactor to facilitate hydrogen transfers in the production of acetyl CoA and ATP. Third, after ATP is produced in the mitochondrial matrix, it carries a negative charge. ATP is then attached to magnesium, and in this stable form, can be mobilized to where it is needed in the capillary cell. Magnesium deficiency will limit ATP mobilization from the mitochondrial matrix, which in the case of the capillary cell, limits the capacity of mitochondria to deliver adequate amounts of energy to outer membranes to support a rigorous active transport of inflammatory mediators into the interstitial space. Without this support, inflammatory breach within the interstitial space is biased to become chronic, thereby creating the initial crack of the door allowing for a chronic inflammatory interstitial space agenda and the eventual coalescence of the inflammatory matrix.

With so much at stake involving magnesium, it becomes imperative that magnesium levels in the blood be checked in high risk situations and supplemented when low. The spiral of magnesium deficiency not only impacts capillary and endothelial cells but expands to also include the homeostasis of the interstitial space and the end organ it serves.

Magnesium is currently FDA approved to treat magnesium deficiency and is also used for the treatment of certain heart arrhythmias, constipation, and certain pregnancy complications. Some magnesium products, like magnesium citrate, can cause diarrhea and interfere with the absorption of other medications. Switching magnesium products from magnesium oxide to magnesium malate, glycinate, taurate or gluconate can improve absorption and reduce side effects without necessarily escalating the dose. In lieu of magnesium supplements, the Mediterranean diet contains high concentrations of magnesium and could be used as a supplement replacement.

Summary
Magnesium is an essential mineral integrally involved in cellular mitochondrial energy production and transport. Lower levels of blood

plasma magnesium make the interstitial spaces more susceptible to chronic inflammation by impairing delivery of energy from mitochondria to capillary cell outer membranes to facilitate active transport processes. Chronic inflammation is then afforded opportunity to build momentum within the interstitial space. The long-term repercussions from chronic magnesium deficiency make chronic inflammation within the interstitial space more likely which would eventually lead to the coalescing of the inflammatory matrix, pirating of the capillary cell outer membranes and subsequent anti-organ disease state venues.

Antioxidants

With advanced age and chronic inflammation in the interstitial spaces of end organs, vascular inflammatory free radicals increase within interstitial spaces, toxic reactive oxygen species (ROS) increase in all cells including capillary cells, and antioxidants decrease in all cells. Antioxidants are biased to decrease from combinations of *reduced* intestinal absorption, *underproduction,* or *overutilization* within a given cell. In capillary cell mitochondria, persistently reduced antioxidant levels are seen with excessive energy production and high concentrations of superoxide exhaust as seen with chronic interstitial space inflammation. As capillary cell antioxidant levels decline (from overutilization and underproduction) the mitochondrial matrix naked DNA is victimized by superoxide cross linkage. With loss of DNA coding instructions, protein synthesis malfunctions. What proteins are synthesized by mitochondria either don't do what's expected or do so poorly. This becomes the primary mechanism of mitochondrial fission, suicide and reduced mitochondrial volumes.

For best results, *antioxidant refurbishment* requires a plant based diet, selected supplementation, reduced interstitial space inflammatory free radical burden, a robust capillary cell dance that includes a back and forth pendulum swing of mitochondrial combustion. This allows antioxidants to re -accumulate without getting exhausted and to function as part of a team of antioxidants to block proinflammatory chain reactions.

There are many different molecules within the human cell that can function as antioxidants. For purposes of discussion the more-common antioxidants found in capillary and endothelial cells include the *glutathione* family (synthesized from the amino acid *cysteine* and *N-acetyl cysteine*), the *MnSOD* family (*manganese superoxide dismutase*), *alpha-lipoic acid (ALA)*, and *vitamins C* and *E family*. As has already been discussed, DHA (along with DHA/PPARs) and coenzyme Q_{10} can also act as antioxidants. With optimal intracellular homeostasis, on-off switches and feedback loops work together to cause checks and balances that preclude free radical chain reactions. In this sense, optimal capillary cell homeostasis produces one large continuous anti-oxidant feedback loop that keeps the capillary cell dancing while sanitizing the interstitial space while nurturing and rejuvenating the end organ.

An antioxidant's *flexibility* to reduce free radicals is based on its concentration, solubility to water or fat and how it teams with other anti-oxidants. Fat-soluble antioxidants are better at crossing cell membranes. Alpha-lipoic acid (ALA), a short-chain omega-3 fatty acid, and coenzyme Q10 are examples of antioxidants that are flexible based on being fat- and water-soluble. ALA can be obtained from ingesting phytonutrients, but it can also be manufactured in liposomes of most cells by breaking down longer chained fatty acids. Like coenzyme Q_{10}, ALA has a dual role of facilitating mitochondrial energy combustion while also neutralizing its free radical exhaust. The teams of vitamins C and E and ALA, as well as MnSOD and glutathione, and then DHA/PPAR and coenzyme Q10, work collaboratively to detoxify emerging sets of free radicals brought about by capillary cell mitochondrial combustion. They can also venture into the capillary cell's cytoplasm and interstitial space to neutralize free radicals when called upon.

Whereas ALA can be produced in liposomes, vitamins C and the vitamin E family must be obtained from ingested nutrient. The vitamin E family is made up of *alpha, delta,* and *gamma* subtypes, all of whom play different roles in free radical management. While most vitamin E supplements contain *alpha tocopherol,* the most antioxidant vitamin E punch may come from *gamma tocopherol.* MnSOD and glutathione antioxidant families are produced within all human cells that contain mitochondria and are integral to neutralizing the residues of mitochondrial energy combustion. Their levels can easily decline when over utilized from chronic energy combustion, which is prevalent with chronic interstitial space inflammation and a blocked capillary cell pivot and swing dance.

Antioxidants routinely decrease too much stress, chronic sleep deprivation, sustained immobility, or abundant interstitial space vascular inflammatory free radicals that include AGEs, LDL cholesterol, triglycerides, alcohol, drugs or tobacco free radicals. Any or all of these proinflammatory lifestyle choices produce chronic inflammation and block capillary cell mitochondrial combustion swinging thereby exhausting antioxidants and creating toxic superoxide free radical lingering within mitochondria. The overworked and exhausted antioxidants within capillary mitochondria become the driving mechanism to damaged DNA, reduction in mitochondrial volumes, pseudocapillarization of outer membrane receptors and the subsequent pirating of them by duped immune arsenal. Anti-organ disease venues are just around the corner.

Supplementing antioxidants to be effective must always be accompanied by reducing vascular inflammatory free radicals within interstitial spaces. Without reducing the vascular inflammatory free radical elephant in the room, mitochondrial combustion will stay stuck in energy and antioxidants will never be adequately refurbished. Pivoting lifestyle choices becomes mandatory for capillary cell outer membranes to downshift a permeability pivot.

Given the fact that antioxidants decline with age and chronic interstitial space inflammation, the argument can be made to supplement them. Dosing guidelines are lacking, however, 500–1,000 mg/day of vitamin C, 400–800 IU/day of a mixed tocopherol (alpha, delta, and gamma vitamin E), 200–400 mg/day of ALA, and 500–600 mg/day of NAC (N-acetyl cysteine, the absorbable cysteine for glutathione production), coupled with coenzyme Q10- 200 mg day and DHA/EPA oils 1-2 gram daily. All of these are reasonably safe to take as these doses and can be adjusted based on prevailing clinical conditions. There is no one dose fits all, and supplementing may not be necessary, if the diet conforms to a Mediterranean diet and lifestyles have conformed to be completely anti-inflammatory. Most need not worry about these supplements if under 50 years of age unless there are special circumstances.

Summary

Increasing endothelial and capillary-cell free-radical (ROS) burden becomes a serious problem with advanced age and chronic interstitial space inflammation. Progressive free radical damage to capillary cell nuclear and mitochondrial DNA depletes mitochondrial volumes. This eventually disrupts outer membrane protein receptors, thereby paving the way for an interstitial space chronic inflammatory coupe of the capillary cell outer membrane. Supplementing antioxidants, coupled with lifestyle adjustments and selected medications to treat already existing anti-organ disease venues, enables capillary cells a chance to restore their dance thereby paving the way towards rejuvenation.

B Vitamins: The *Backbone* to Mitochondrial Function

B vitamins or B complex, as they are collectively labelled, are integral to mitochondrial combustion in all cells, including capillary and endothelial cells. B vitamins are essential vitamins, meaning they have to be ingested and absorbed from nutrient-rich dietary sources. With advanced age and chronic interstitial space inflammation, B vitamin levels trend lower or become less effective in what they do. In those over 50 years of age, supplementing B vitamins while simultaneously reducing proinflammatory behaviors, becomes a simple two step to optimizing both their levels and benefits.

B vitamins facilitate methylated carbon (CH_3) transfers between molecules. For example, in the mitochondrial inner membrane, *vitamin B_9 (folate/folic acid)* facilitates methylated carbon transfers that assist in the passage of electrons through the cytochrome system. Folate is also an essential cofactor in cellular regenerative processes, such as in the replication of mitochondrial DNA. Because of B complex involvement in facilitating both sides of mitochondrial combustion (energy and nitric oxide), they are essential to executing endothelial and capillary cell dual function, rejuvenation, interstitial space sanitation, and optimizing end organ function.

Listed below are the different B vitamins and how they facilitate mitochondrial mechanics:

- B_6 *(pyridoxine)*, B_9 *(folate/folic acid)*, and B_{12} *(cyanocobalamin)* are cofactors that facilitate conversion of methionine/cysteine to glutathione, a potent, all-purpose antioxidant in the mitochondrial matrix.
- B_1 *(thiamine)*, B_2 *(riboflavin)*, B_3 *(niacin)*, B_5 *(pantothenic acid)*, and B_6 *(pyridoxine)* are required as cofactors for the Krebs cycle.
- B_2 *(riboflavin)* and B_9 *(folate/folic acid)* are required for movement of electrons through the cytochrome system of the mitochondrial inner membrane.
- B_3 *(niacin)* is required to make nicotinamide adenine dinucleotide (NAD) from nicotinamide riboside (NR). NAD transports hydrogen to the electron transport chain to produce energy. Niacin is also used in the production of *nicotinamide adenine dinucleotide phosphate (NADPH)*, which is used to transfer hydrogen in the production of nitric oxide (see figure 17 in the appendix).
- B_9 *(folate/folic acid)* facilitates mitochondrial membrane repair and DNA replication.

For most older -adults, it is safe and inexpensive to take a B-complex vitamin daily. Although B-complex is well tolerated, there are no approved FDA indications. There can be occasional side effects that are usually dose related and include nausea, flushing, dizziness, rash, or itching. Taking a B-complex tablet with food or a baby aspirin eliminates most side effects. Just like any supplement, there are multiple vendors selling them. It is wise to choose a company with a good reputation for quality.

Summary

Individual B vitamins have been approved to treat certain medical conditions, including chronic alcoholism and alcohol withdrawal (thiamine and folic acid), anemia (when from deficiencies of folic acid or cyanocobalamin), as well as elevated blood plasma homocysteine (pyridoxine and folic acid, with or without cyanocobalamin), and LDL cholesterol levels (niacin). When the B complex of vitamins are supplemented by older adults, they improve efficiency of mitochondrial combustion when it swings to either energy or nitric oxide. They are more effective when chronic inflammatory interstitial space influences are concomitantly reduced.

Mitochondrial "Basic Materials"

To facilitate a robust energy and nitric oxide combustion, capillary-cell mitochondria must have a full complement of *basic raw materials* that include energy substrate (pyruvate, fatty acids), oxygen, phosphorus, iron, calcium, magnesium, manganese, sodium, potassium, citrulline, arginine, cysteine, and lysine. Deficiencies of raw materials are more common with highly processed "empty calorie" western diets and can result in erratic and uneven mitochondrial combustion in all cells. This can sometimes make the difference to chronic inflammation being able to establish an interstitial space foothold.

A very important and often overlooked step in mitochondrial combustion involves the *N-acetylation* of energy substrates to make acetyl CoA, which becomes the hub of energy and nitric oxide combustion. N-acetylation requires the *amino acid- lysine*, which facilitates the stripping of carbon from pyruvate and fatty acids to make *acetyl coenzyme A (acetyl CoA)*. Once lysine has facilitated conversion to acetyl CoA, it is mobilized to the Krebs cycle (energy combustion), where hydrogen is stripped from it and carried to the cytochromes, or it is shuttled to ribosomes or rough endoplasmic reticulum, to facilitate protein synthesis (nitric oxide combustion).

Summary

Most basic materials that are essential for mitochondrial combustion are abundant in fresh vegetables, such as green leafy varieties, cabbage, chard, broccoli, asparagus, spinach, kale, and onion. Advanced age, nutrient-poor diets, and chronic inflammation increase risk for deficient mitochondrial raw materials. Deficiency states can be largely resolved by eating plant based nutrient. Eating lightly cooked cruciferous vegetables is a better way of obtaining mitochondrial raw materials than supplementing the individual sums of their parts.

Herbs

Most *edible herbs* can be classified as *superfoods*. Coupled with a diet pivot away from empty-calories, adding herbs to fresh produce cascades additional anti-inflammatory benefits to endothelial and capillary cells by:

- *trickling the pace* of carbohydrate metabolism in the liver, thereby reducing blood sugar surges, adipose buildup and increased blood plasma AGEs, LDL cholesterol and triglyceride levels
- selecting a more optimal intestinal microbiome that improves absorption of nutrient and reduces leaky gut
- providing abundant antioxidants and minerals
- producing specific added-on value to reduce specific proinflammatory risks, such as allicin in garlic to lower LDL cholesterol)

Herbs can be easily grown in most gardens, are often resistant to drought, animals, birds, and insects, and do not require large spaces. Fresh herbs have a higher nutritional value than those that have been processed and dried. Alternatively, most herbs have been conveniently dosed and placed in pills, capsules or flakes, to be taken as supplements or used in cooking. These expensive conveniences come with a price, as processing leaches out much of their vitamin, mineral and fiber content.

Edible herbs can be found in the form of flowers, leaves, stalks, or roots and even in different tree barks. Ingestible herb flowers include arugula, basil, borage, chive (onion or garlic), lavender, orchid, rose, pansy, and snapdragon. Herbs that can be eaten as leaves and stalks include chamomile, chives, cilantro, thyme, dill, parsley, lemon balm, basil, marjoram, oregano, sage, spearmint, peppermint, tarragon, and garlic. Edible herb roots include ginger and turmeric.

Different herbs can produce different anti-inflammatory benefits, all of which suppress chronic interstitial space inflammation and bias upticks in the capillary cell dance. Besides the potent anti-inflammatory effects of allicin, ginger and turmeric roots also provide multipronged anti-inflammatory benefits that produce resistance to anti-organ venues. Because of these anti-inflammatory benefits they must be used with caution when taking traditional medicines, as they can alter their effects. For example, taking a daily baby aspirin or other blood thinner, with fish oil, garlic chives, ginkgo biloba or ginger root, could increase bleeding risk.

Like vegetables, herbs preferably should be consumed fresh rather than prepackaged. The benefits of eating a fresh garlic chives or clove, may be 80% more valuable as compared to taking a capsule or sprinkling flakes of dried herb from a container. If attempting to maximize their anti-inflammatory benefits, they should be used regularly, and preferably hand -picked from a well cultivated garden.

Summary

Most edible herbs preserve the capillary cell dance by abundantly supplying essential vitamins, minerals and nutrient while also reducing vascular inflammatory free radicals within interstitial spaces. When coupled with other behaviors that further reduce vascular inflammatory free radical interstitial space seeding, they provide anti-inflammatory momentum that drives optimal capillary cell homeostasis. The cascades that follow include a line in the sand demarcation of anti-organ interstitial space influence. As such, the consistent use of herbs improve end organ function, reduce pain and fatigue, block the spread and progression of chronic illnesses, and as such, become an antidote to aging.

Therapeutic Conclusions

Reviving capillary and endothelial cells throughout the arterial tree from chronic interstitial-space inflammation becomes the essential pivot to resuscitating vitality in all end-organs. Revival is greatly benefitted from the generous use of herbs. When combined with intentional lifestyle changes, supplements, and selected medicinals, the foundation for an all –out assault on anti-organ mechanics is created. Anti-inflammatory momentum is generated to enable capillary cells to come back from being blind sighted by chronic interstitial space inflammatory deception. If they can reestablish their footing and resume the fluxing and swinging of outer membrane permeability and mitochondrial combustion, they stand a chance to rejuvenate. The anti-inflammatory momentum parlays remissions to serious anti-organ venues that subsequently improve end organ function and reduced fatigue and pain. The key to good health requires the capillary cell take back control of the interstitial space.

As the anti-organ goes into solitary confinement and the capillary cell remerges as the guardian of the interstitial space, chronic inflammatory anti-organ venues get sacked. When immune arsenal and mesenchymal cells reestablish allegiance to the capillary cell- end organ axis, interstitial space scarring can reverse, cancer cells and infectious agents once again become targeted for removal, and thrombosis risk becomes unhinged. Nagging health issues, such as achy joints, brain fog (or progressive dementia), exertional fatigue and sexual dysfunction remit to levels not seen for decades.

It's okay to be a skeptic about reversing anti-inflammatory momentum. I would be too if I was trying to digest all of this for the first time. It is a stretch for many to connect reducing the chronic inflammatory dots to disease treatment and prevention, let alone all the other anti-inflammatory fall-out that follows. But unlike disease treatment models, where expensive surgeries, interventions, chemotherapies, surveillance and imaging become a prison, reducing chronic inflammatory influences within interstitial spaces through lifestyle adjustments becomes an uplifting life- giving *Rejuvenation*. The renewal releases life exuberance rather than shackles it. It is time to set sail on a different horizon to claim victory over fatigue and pain. Your essence need not become isolated or hidden but rather can come out from behind the shadow cast by chronic inflammatory anesthesia.

Chapter 9

THE FINAL EXAM

Dodging an imminent heart attack and having a stent placed in the widow-maker of coronary arteries at age fifty-four was more than a sobering wake- up call. Upon reflection it should not have been unexpected. My life for quite some time had gone on some kind of proinflammatory autopilot and I, like most in midlife, had succumbed to a reactive lifestyle filled with stress, sleep deprivation, knee jerk comfort food eating and weight gain. What made all of this even worse was the forgone conclusion that at age 50 plus, I was bulletproof. As long as I did most things in moderation, I would kick my genetic ticking time bombs of premature heart attacks and strokes to the curb. After all, I was not my father or grandfather. I really never smoked and they did. Case closed. I would be okay. I could ignore all the budding inflammatory red flags of the cholesterol and blood pressure creep, because it could not possibly happen to me. Denial worked—or at least it did until I was staring at a coffin.

Unbeknownst to me, at age 54 as I ignored the inflammatory red flags and ground out a living as a doctor working 12 hour days, I was already in a deep medical hole. It was just a matter of time, maybe weeks to months, and it would have been over. In spite of weight gain, poor sleep, excessive stress, and the proverbial midlife blood pressure and LDL cholesterol creep, I went on as if nothing was happening to me. In other words, vascular inflammatory free radical warning shots were buzzing all around me and I chose not to see or hear them. Sound familiar?

After a fortuitous series of events occurred, and a coronary stent was placed in my nearly blocked coronary artery, I came home with a swollen right groin and a bruised psyche. For weeks I went back into time in attempts to work out my denial. What emerged was shocking. I had invented a denial system that protected me from having to honestly answer what I was doing to myself.

Slowly these denial layers were unraveled and changes were made. Certain changes were easier to make than others. The hardest was letting go of my 24-7 on call availability for most hospital emergencies. This created large amount of stress that I routinely underestimated, not to mention the numerous night calls and sleep deprivation that went with it. This is where I should have listened to my wife but didn't. Adjusting was a process, but giving up the stress and sleep deprivation of hospital work was a stubborn last item to turn over. Happily I made adjustments in everything else until one fateful day the inability to limit hospital work came back to haunt and almost kill me.

"Help! I'm over here!" I shouted hoarsely, gasping with all the reserve that I had left.

I was laying semi -upright with my upper body propped by the sloping hillside underneath a dried-out, prickly shrub. I could hear muffled voices from over my right shoulder, accompanied by the rustling of dried out brush. I was too dizzy and weak to stand or wave, let alone walk. My head pounded with pain and my chest had a deep ache on the right side that made deep breathing impossible. As I gazed down at my hands, my fingers were numb, barely moveable, with at least one grossly deformed. Both wrists looked detached from my arm. Blood was dripping profusely from my forehead, and I was unable to turn my head to the right because of pressure in my neck.

It was late June afternoon and the sun was just beginning to hide behind mountain peaks, causing the air to quickly cool. I was getting cold, in fact, shivering. Realizing I could not move and with no cell phone reception I had one option; hunker down and hope someone, anyone would come after me.

As it turned out, I had gone hiking alone. A late-morning emergent call and visit to the hospital caused me to miss meeting up with a seven-member hiking group. When I finally arrived at the starting point, about 45 minutes late, they were long gone. I made the assumption that I could catch them and set out walking at fast pace.

As I hiked deeper into the wilderness while following a stream, the trail narrowed and forked into two directions. Three hours into the hike, the fork forced me to make a directional choice. I chose to go right, while unbeknownst to me, my hiking group went left.

Hiking perhaps a half mile further it was now 3 PM. I found a place to sit, eat lunch, and soak my feet in the cold stream of mountain-water. As I sat there, I let my thoughts wander. For a moment, I was care-free and completely relaxed, but then with a chill in the air caused by a shadow from the setting sun hiding behind a mountain top, and I knew I should head back.

As I gathered my shoes and hiking gear, I heard garbled and faint voices downstream from where I had previously hiked. I yelled as loud as I could but got no response, thinking this was my hiking group. Disappointed, I realized that I would be hiking back alone, again. I started my way back down the mountain, again following the stream. On the way back down, I chose not to rock hop the stream, preferring to keep my feet dry and reduce risk for a slip on wet stones. This meant having to climb rugged and often virgin terrain in order to circumvent the moving water of the stream.

About 20 minutes in, with one step on loose soil over a steep cavern, I fell at an angle, headfirst, for about twenty feet. Slowly regaining consciousness and gathering myself over the next 30 minutes or so, I waited under the scrub until the voices were heard.

"I'm over here!" I shouted again and again.

The voices got closer.

I yelped more.

"Over here! Over here! Over here!"

A few moments later, in what felt like an eternity, I was spotted!

Four adults—two men and two women—had noticed my baseball cap in the dense shrubbery, which had fallen off from the fall. Within minutes, they went to work. After assessing injuries, they had my head straddled, wounds bandaged, and plans made get me out of there. The two women would stay, and the two men would rock hop down the stream for more help. What made this different was that my rescuers were actually elite hikers with extensive experience. The two men had advanced survival training in the United States military and all four were in excellent shape. As luck would have it they choose the same path down the mountain as I had. They could just as easily have chosen to rock hop or alternatively hike the opposite side of the stream.

In less than an hour, I could hear the approaching clatter of a helicopter propeller. Soon, a young man, fit and perhaps in his mid to late-twenties, harnessed down from the hovering helicopter, assessed my injuries, and then advised me to harness and be lifted up to the helicopter rather than use a stretcher.

I went with his recommendation. With ample assistance from the two nightingales, I staggered to stand and was then strapped into the vertical harness and pulled about ninety feet into the air. From there, I dangled for a while until my left arm was grabbed. In one motion, I was hoisted onto the backseat of the helicopter where I plopped down in a thud, not to move again until the helicopter landed.

Further resuscitation was then implemented. As I was being questioned, vital signs were recorded, oxygen was shoved up my nose, an intravenous line was started in my arm, and a morphine injection was given. Within a few minutes, I was being jettisoned towards the setting sun.

The thud of the helicopter landing on the roof of the hospital quickly changed the ambiance. As the helicopter door flew open, I was greeted by a bustling array of people chirping anxiously about how to get me on the awaiting gurney. After extrication from the helicopter, I took a short bumpy ride to an elevator which deposited me into a crowded, well lit, but noisy trauma room. I was quickly stripped of my clothing, strapped onto a noisy monitoring system, and connected to IV drips. For the next three hours, X-ray and imaging studies came one after another, as I was reassessed, sutured and bandaged.

After about four hours in the trauma room, I learned that I had broken at least fourteen different bones and would need non emergent surgery. I left the trauma room to a monitored hospital bed with bulky arm casts, a finger splint, a compressed face as a result of an orbital fracture, and several stitches to my chin. I had a partial collapse of my left lung, several rib fractures, air going up into my neck form a punctured lung and kidney injury from the leaking of muscle enzymes. In spite of all this, my vital signs remained stable.

Within 12 hours the lungs had re expanded, the air in my neck had departed, and the kidney function had reverted back to normal. At midmorning an orthopedic surgeon walked in, closed the curtain, and introduced himself.

"Good morning. Let me take a look at your wrists." After a brief glimpse at the bulky casts, he eyeballed my hands and asked if I had sensation and could move my fingers. After responding affirmatively, he made mention of more wrist imaging and then said that surgery would be scheduled for my wrists and face the following day. He left quickly, before I had enough where withal to muster a question from my still groggy brain. Having next day surgery to fix my orthopedic problems on the next day given all my trauma complications was unexpected. Did lifestyle adjustments pave the way for this quick reversal and extensive next day surgery under general anesthesia? What else was I to think?

By 10 o'clock the next morning, I was in the surgery holding area, where I met the anesthesiologist. As he started an IV in my foot, he casually asked me about my medical history which included my previous coronary stent. On the basis of my overall health, the decision had been made to schedule me for one five-hour surgery with multiple fix procedures rather than break it up into two different surgeries. One surgery could have more anesthetic risk but would enable a faster post-op recovery. This became another sign, that even compromised from multiple trauma, known coronary artery disease and recovering kidney and lung function, my body was judged capable of handling a single more demanding surgery.

After five plus hours of surgery, I emerged from induced coma in the recovery room, with a full cast on my left arm, an external metal fixator brace on my right forearm, and a bulky dressing on my face. It was over, and I was told things could not have gone better—or so I thought. There were no intraoperative complications, and after a couple of hours in the recovery area, I was brought back to my hospital room.

Then the second nightmare emerged.

My arm suddenly felt like it had been cut off. The pain coming from my right shoulder was excruciating, by far the worst I had every felt. My desperate screams of "Help me! Help me! The pain is killing me!" fell on deaf ears.

Minutes passed, and still no response.

It turned out that post-op orders did not include pain medicine. The change of shift had compounded the delay. I was being tortured from excruciating pain and had no way out.

After several minutes of screaming, the intravenous pain injection was finally given and I mercifully settled down. I should have had a heart attack right then. Instead, even with all that pain, the heart monitor remained steady without one missed beat. Remarkably, the pain blitz caused no collateral damage. At this point I had more than enough reason for my heart to sputter but it didn't. More points for lifestyle adjustment.

At 2:00 a.m. the first post- operative night, I awoke from a light slumber to visual hallucinations and a dull but substantial pressure ache in my lower abdomen. At that moment I could not recall when I last urinated, let alone when I last played pong, which is what the up and down motion of television screen reminded me of.

It was again major decision time. I summoned the nurse, and began to negotiate a narcotic truce, knowing that it was contributing to both my obstructed bladder and visual hallucinations. We agreed to stop the IV narcotic drip in exchange for taking an oral pain pill plus a periodic intravenous injection of a non- narcotic pain reliever. In addition I was not to receive a bladder catheter unless I cried uncle. The bet was, that taking away the narcotic infusion, I would eliminate the hallucinations and unblock my bladder just enough to where I could squirt urine out of my distended bladder.

At about 3:00 a.m., I grabbed the urinal with my barely functioning finger tips, and once again bore down. Out squirted a tablespoon of urine. Success! From then on, every 5 minutes or so, bearing down yielded additional squirts of urine into the urinal, with each one yielding a bit more than the previous squirt. I had bypassed a major post op bullet. The catheter into my bladder could have set back my recovery for days, let alone the risk for a bladder infection. In addition, the hallucinations quickly resolved. Now all I had to do was figure out how to use pain medications to control the surgical pain emanating from the right arm.

The following day was Wednesday, the first postoperative day and the third day in the hospital. To be discharged I now needed to accomplish three things; suitable pain management, the ability to independently transfer from a bed to chair, and the capacity to urinate and defecate. Physical therapists came by and had me transferring and walking the hallway with a walker by mid -afternoon. But what would going to the bathroom look like with two disabled and casted arms?

At 10 AM I asked for MOM (also known as milk of magnesia). In early afternoon after lunch, I got up out of bed and took my chances going to the bathroom. As I sat and bore down I did not feel confident of getting something accomplished. On the second try, with persistence, a BM. Wiping was next to impossible but I found a way. By 4 PM with all criteria met, I requested discharge for the following morning. The staff marginalized my request but I persisted. They in essence said that my discharge was days premature, especially for a nearly 60 year old man with the extent of injury and surgery that I had.

On Thursday morning, I was discharged home. Three and one half days after a twenty-foot fall, fourteen broken bones, a collapsed lung, a skull and orbital fracture, kidney failure, and air in my neck, not to mention a 5 hours of surgery, a pain management snafu, visual hallucinations and urinary retention, I was discharged! Coincidental? I think not.

Within a few days of being home, I was actively stretching and moving my arms in all directions. After three weeks, I celebrated my 59th birthday with an early morning walk around the neighborhood and taking my stick shift jeep to the office to do paper work. At five weeks, with the left arm cast and right arm external fixator removed, and off all pain management, I was now receiving hand physical therapy, managing hospital patients and seeing a full complement of office patients.

Six years later, I have *no residual effects* from the fall or treatment. In fact, I feel better today than I did before the fall happened.

So what is the point? All the brokered hospital gambits aside, neither the speed nor comprehensiveness of recovery would have been possible without the capillary cell's capacity to dance, manage and restore the interstitial spaces of all the traumatized end organs, and that lifestyle adjustments made in the previous four years were primarily responsible. With the capillary cells effectively dancing and eliciting appropriate immune responses into the interstitial spaces of severely traumatized end organs, healing was faster and with less scarring. In a strange sense, the fall and multi -end organ blunt trauma assault followed by a complete and rapid recovery, became a *final exam* as to how effective the capillary cell dance had actually become. Through lifestyle adjustments, one prescription medication and supplements, vascular inflammatory free-radical seeds had been reduced, and chronic inflammatory influences within interstitial spaces diminished, to where capillary cell rejuvenation had occurred. The rejuvenated endothelial and capillary cells of the entire vascular tree enabled a quicker and more comprehensive recovery.

In retrospect, I made a serious hiking mistake. I should not have hiked alone. But the outcome could have been much worse without a little bit of luck and an endothelial- and capillary-cell network prepared to initiate proper healing cascades. Lifestyle matters, and in my case, it just might have saved my life.

Chapter 10

THE CAPILLARY-CELL PIVOT AND PENDULUM-SWING DANCE: GROUND ZERO FOR ANTIAGING

Aging and chronic interstitial space inflammation stagnate capillary cell outer membrane permeability to eventually doom the cell to futility. Antiaging is linked to a rigorous back and forth fluxing of capillary cell outer membrane permeability. Anti-inflammatory lifestyles, coupled with what I would call functional medicinals and supplements, interrupt chronic interstitial space inflammation to subsequently slow or reverse aging by enabling the return of the capillary cell outer membrane permeability pivot and mitochondrial combustion swing, which I have called the capillary cell dance.

Capillary cell dancing becomes the penultimate anti-inflammatory feedback loop. By creating a back and forth rhythm to capillary cell outer membrane permeability and mitochondrial combustion of energy and nitric oxide, cascading feedback loops feed off of this dance to induce an optimal homeostasis that enables capillary cells to sanitize the interstitial space, optimize on demand end organ function while stemming and pacing their own rejuvenation as well as that of its interstitial space partners, the mesenchymal and end organ cells. Within the capillary cell, the feedback relationships between on-off switches, gluconeogenesis, glycolysis, and mitochondrial combustion, as well as antioxidant balance and maintenance, are all on short leashes based on a rhythmic check and balance system tied to their dance.

When capillaries are dancing, chronic interstitial space inflammation is tamed, mesenchymal and immune arsenal are squarely encamped into the capillary cell fold, anti-organ venues are laid to rest, and the chronic disease popups linked to thrombotic- hypoxic -ischemia, rogue autoimmune complexes, infections, cancer and scarring become bad santas once removed. The instigators for or against the capillary cell dance begins with vascular inflammatory free radicals harbored within the interstitial space. The persistence of too many and the capillary cell cannot muster enough immune support from blood plasma and elsewhere to defend against them. Therein is the beginning seed to chronic inflammation.

What this discussion implies is that classic disease treatment is a late stage treatment, where chronic inflammation has matured to a level where it has coalesced elements within the interstitial space to form an anti-organ with disease venues. Disease is being treated after the anti-organ has essentially nullified normal immune processes and what's more, is using them to its own benefit. Disease treatment, while attacking the disease(s) the anti -organ has brokered, does little to stem other anti-organ venues or address the elephant in the room- the root cause(s)of chronic inflammation and anti –organ preeminence. As a result, one disease process occurs after another, often seeming disjointed and unrelated, as different end organ s are picked off with anti-organ interstitial space venues.

In contrast to disease treatment, which is a relentless, never ending and expensive circle of tests, treatments, surgeries, and interventions, followed by more tests and treatments, *wellness gets off this runaway train and focuses on root causes of inflammation,* which as this book amply demonstrates, is several steps in front of disease treatment. Attacking the root causes of inflammation first, rather than last or not at all, puts the onus back on our own natural immunity to halt the inflammatory process before it progresses.

Without doing so, chronic inflammation is allowed to fester. This leads to an interstitial pace breeding ground, a several step progression of chronic inflammatory maturation that includes the evolution of an inflammatory matrix and the shutting down of the capillary cell dance. This is followed by a relentless assault on capillary cell integrity that includes in block reduction of capillary cell mitochondria, loss of outer membrane receptors, voltage gradients and pore diversity (pseudocapillarization), and then the coup de tat pirating of capillary cell outer membrane receptors by duped immune arsenal. After all these transitional steps, all that is left is for the anti-organ to step into the interstitial space and choose which sets of disease inducing venues to implement.

By addressing vascular inflammatory free radicals first, downstream disease processes are brought to their knees even before they have even started to form. This creates a different kind of health care momentum that promotes wellness and postpones indefinitely downstream anti-organ chronic illnesses and the waves of fatigue and pain they generate. The key to wellness is to absolutely drop kick vascular inflammatory free radicals, by any means possible, before they can affront the capillary cell dance.

Plain and simple, an accent on vegetable-based eating, daily exercise, intentional stress mediation, while limiting sleep deprivation, halts chronic inflammation. In some, this will not likely be enough. Diets may have to be further restricted, exercise more refined, and the use of medicinals and supplements may be required. All of this to block chronic interstitials pace inflammation and enable the capillary cells to pivot and swing dance.

In this model of wellness, behaviors become more important than drugs, surgeries and interventions. All *behaviors, medicines, and supplements* we choose, should by- intention, be viewed as either pro- or anti-inflammatory to our interstitial spaces. From this perspective, the priorities of good health are not based on access to drugs, surgery and imaging but rather the choices we make in every-day life. Bad choices cause bad outcomes that involve anti-organ venues. Wellness assumes that epigenetics can trump bad genetics, but bad behaviors trump everything else.

When we choose to implement anti-inflammatory behaviors, we are choosing to consciously reduce interstitial space vascular inflammatory free radicals. Doing so reduces interstitial space *inflammatory mediator burden* which affords the adjoining capillary cell a better chance of nullifying existing free radicals within the interstitial space. Resolution enables the endothelial and capillary cell to downshift their permeability, as they no longer need energy to mobilize additional immune arsenal into the interstitial space. This pivot, produces a powerful feedback loop that pushes the pendulum swinging of mitochondrial combustion to nitric oxide. Nitric oxide shifts capillary cell purpose from interstitial space sanitation to end organ enrichment and rejuvenation of its own infrastructure, mitochondrial volumes and outer membrane receptors. Similar rejuvenation is paced reciprocally to the end organ as well. The capillary cell dance becomes the vehicle of *rejuvenation and wellness*. When the dance is brisk, not only is capillary cell homeostasis optimized, but chronic inflammation is severely handicapped, meaning there is no chance for chronic inflammatory repercussions involving the inflammatory matrix or anti-organ.

The rejuvenation that occurs from within the shadows of capillary cell mitochondrial nitric oxide combustion becomes nature's built in *fountain of youth*, as it reinvigorates interstitial space immune surveillance while optimally supporting end-organ functional mechanics. The feedback-loop crisscrossing of capillary and end-organ outer-membrane permeability and mitochondrial combustion seals their mutual intimacy.

The bullets below summarize the pitch battle for control of the interstitial spaces between endothelial and capillary cells and chronic inflammation. The winner gets enormous influence over the space. The anti-inflammatory cascades that accompany the capillary cell should it win out are as follows:

- Vascular inflammatory free radical festering is neutralized. Capillary cell fluxing of permeability persists or returns, and is accompanied by the back and forth swinging of mitochondrial combustion. Capillary cells are dancing!

- Anti-organ venues are either blocked or never get access to the interstitial space. These include different assortments of interstitial space fibrous scar and amyloid deposition, cancer growth, infections, autoimmune diseases, and thrombotic-hypoxic-ischemic events and all the mosaics of different diseases that can be attributable to them.

- Within all endothelial and end organ cells, energy substrate utilization improves. This reduces insulin resistance, AGEs, LDL cholesterol and triglyceride levels, among others in the blood. Included in this homeostasis is a bias against gluconeogenesis and towards more pyruvate utilization in mitochondrial combustion.

- With improved interstitial space sanitation, passive diffusion of gases through membrane surfaces improves. This means that more oxygen and carbon dioxide get to where they are supposed to go more efficiently. This makes end organs and their mitochondria more responsive to on demand changes in capacity to make energy to support their specific function.

- Endothelial and capillary cell mitochondrial nitric oxide combustion becomes restorative thereby sealing improved future function to itself and its partners.

- Restoring capillary cell outer membrane receptors and mitochondrial volumes pays forward the future precise and targeted management of interstitial space inflammatory breach. This makes future interstitial space chronic inflammation less likely.

- These cellular outcomes that enable capillary cell dancing induce antiaging effects that also block pain, fatigue and chronic illness.

Making poor lifestyle choices doubles down inflammation as we get older. A forty year-old obese diabetic, who also smokes a daily pack of cigarettes, has unleashed so much chronic interstitial space inflammation that he or she feel, thinks and moves more like an eighty-year-old. An eighty-five-year-old, who exercises regularly, eats a vegetable rich diet rich, sleeps continuously for seven hours each night, and is not stress encumbered, has tame interstitial space inflammation and moves and feels more like a forty-year-old. We can choose correctly and stay relevant or we can live addicted and reactional and die decades before we should have to.

There are no shortcuts, silver bullets, or magic pills to achieving the capillary and endothelial cell dance. If we approach chronic inflammation with gimmicks they will backfire. Knee-jerk use of prescription medications to chronic inflammatory red flags such as insomnia, pain, anxiety and fatigue will not necessarily help remove the chronic inflammatory interstitial space impetus and may contribute to more addictions and proinflammatory behaviors. Without a meaningful lifestyle overhaul that affronts root causes of chronic inflammation, the interstitial space game is over before it starts. Band aid approaches enable anti-organ venues and the inevitable requirement for disease treatment and the encirclement of the medical industrial complex. While these treatments are necessary and well intentioned, they could all have been largely prevented or postponed with some simple steps taken earlier in the course of chronic inflammatory progression.

Strategies that eliminate chronic inflammation, from whatever cause, headline wellness and should be established well before disease treatment is even on the table. Transitioning to more exercise, and harvesting home grown vegetables, while eliminating tobacco, sugars, trans- fats, most salt, alcohol, addictive sleep aids, narcotic pain pills, and street drugs should occur sooner rather than later. All this gets complicated, when chronic inflammation unleashes waves of pain and fatigue.

Pain management can become a can of worms when the focus is symptom rather than inflammation management. Focus on symptomatic pain management, while initially important, if not pivoted to anti-inflammatory management will spiral addictions to pain drugs or cause bleeding and hypertension from others. This same principle can be applied to treatment of insomnia or anxiety. Symptom treatment, unless transitioned to anti-inflammatory treatment results in addictions that cascade to other bad habits. As providers in the front lines we must have the courage to anticipate the different outcomes, and adjust care to wellness when it comes to managing pain, fatigue, insomnia or anxiety. The disease treatment model has had its place in the sun for the last few centuries, but it now must a least share some of the limelight with wellness. Without doing so, none of us will be able to afford disease treatment much longer moving forward.

Targeted medicinal treatments, particularly when preexisting anti-organ venues have established a foothold, are often essential to recouping capillary cell control of the interstitial space. When coupled with supplements, the combination enables capillary cells to re- find their footing and reestablish their dance. When done thoughtfully and with added lifestyle integration, capillary cell recovery can be robust leading to brisk outer membrane fluxing and a more rigorous rejuvenation.

Reducing vascular inflammatory free radicals by lifestyle, or if necessary by medications, becomes a root-cause method of reducing risk for chronic interstitial space inflammation. We can choose to live hungover in different disease states and as prisoners to pain and fatigue, or we can choose to unshackle and live without chronic inflammatory encumbrances. Resist the dark path, push back on chronic inflammation and anti-organ emergence, and you can emerge with vitally you never knew was possible. Don't let chronic inflammation become your interstitial space master. Choose wisely, and as capillary-cells dance, so will you. The fountain of youth is not a place but a dance. The time to pivot and *swing rejuvenation* is now!

Glossary

abluminal: The space opposite the luminal side of the capillary and endothelial cell. The abluminal side of the capillary cell is lined by both the continuous outer and basement membranes. Just outside the capillary- or endothelial-cell *basement membrane* lies the *interstitial space* and end-organ epithelial cells. This space is where inflammation occurs that can affect end-organ (in the case of capillary cells) and smooth-muscle function (in the case of endothelial cells of larger arteries).

abscess: A serious infection, usually from bacteria, that can occur in the *interstitial space* of any end organ to seriously compromise its function. Abscess formation can be linked to reduced capillary-cell capacity to perform immune surveillance to the end organ involved, increases in prevalence with chronic increases in vascular inflammatory free radicals, and becomes more common in those who have diabetes or smoke cigarettes.

acetyl coenzyme A (acetyl CoA): The hub of mitochondrial matrix metabolism. In capillary and endothelial cells, pyruvate, fatty acids, and ketone bodies are metabolized to acetyl CoA. Acetyl CoA can then be utilized by the Krebs cycle to increase energy combustion, or it can be diverted and utilized to synthesize proteins and relocate mitochondria to replenish their volumes in the capillary cell.

actin-myosin sliding (muscle contraction): Actin and myosin filaments (in muscle) or fibrils (in capillary cells) utilize energy (ATP) and calcium ions to slide on each other. When a group of actin-myosin filaments slide in unison, muscle contracts. Actin-myosin sliding can increase or decrease, causing both the force and rate of muscle contraction to vary, and is dependent on the volume of ATP provided by mitochondria (muscle tone) and the thickness of the actin-myosin filaments. With aging, actin-myosin filaments thin, causing skeletal-muscle atrophy (also known as *sarcopenia*).

active transport: Refers to membrane transport processes that require energy to move constituent from one side of the membrane to the other. The surge in energy required to service capillary-cell outer-membrane active transport often comes from mitochondria. Active-transport mechanisms through capillary cells include endocytosis, transcellular transport by vesicles and channels, and opening the orifice of the gap junction through actin-myosin fibril contraction. Active transport is utilized to mobilize inflammatory mediators (white blood cells, cytokines) through capillary-cell outer membranes in response to vascular inflammatory free-radical seeds in the interstitial space. *Passive transport* is the opposite, where movement of gases and simple molecules requires no energy or specialized transport vehicles to cross membranes. An example of passive transport would be gas exchange of oxygen and carbon dioxide.

adenosine diphosphate (ADP): This is the energy precursor to *adenosine triphosphate* (ATP). The capillary, endothelial, and almost all other somatic cells utilize the ATP/ADP ratio in the cell's cytoplasm as a strong feedback-loop signal to increase or decrease mitochondrial energy combustion. As ratios decrease, energy combustion increases. This is typically seen when there is chronic inflammation in the interstitial space of end organs and capillary-cell outer membranes are requiring more energy (increased permeability) to move additional inflammatory mediators (white blood cells, cytokines, etc.) into the interstitial space.

adenosine triphosphate (ATP): The basic energy unit of all cells, made from ADP (*adenosine diphosphate*) precursor. ATP can be produced with oxygen (aerobic—in mitochondria) or without oxygen (anaerobic [glycolysis]—in cytoplasm). Utilizing oxygen to make ATP in the mitochondria allows for a much more abundant and efficient source of energy production, and also allows cells to manage surges of energy demand more effectively. Making ATP in mitochondria requires oxygen, ADP, phosphorus, hydrogen, and the enzyme ATP synthetase. By-products of ATP oxidation include carbon dioxide, water, and free radicals, such as superoxide. By-products of glycolysis include lactic acid (lactate).

adipose: Adipose tissue (a group of fat cells) can increase by replication of fat cells, which increases their volume or number, or by hypertrophy, which increases their cellular size. Under duress, liver cells (*hepatocytes*) and skeletal-muscle cells can convert to adipose cells.

adrenaline: A fight-or-flight hormone produced primarily in the adrenal glands and increased with stress or chronic insomnia. When chronically increased from stress or insomnia, it becomes an inflammatory mediator, increasing insulin resistance, blood pressure, and heart rate.

advanced glycation end products (AGEs): Often caused by consuming abundant simple sugars, AGEs act as simple-sugar free radicals in the bloodstream. They attach to membrane proteins without enzymes and cause dysfunction, and also attract more inflammatory mediators to cause additional inflammation.

aerobic exercise: Refers to *continuous-movement exercise,* as opposed to *interrupted-movement exercise* (also known as *anaerobic exercise* or *weight training*). Aerobic exercise has multiple vascular benefits, including increased skeletal-muscle mitochondrial volumes (increased muscle tone), reduced blood pressure, improved weight management, reduced blood sugars, increased sleep quality, and optimized blood lipid profiles. Anaerobic exercise maintains skeletal-muscle mass and bone, tendon, and ligament integrity, thereby optimizing lean body mass and increasing metabolism to burn calories.

aerobic respiration: A term used to define the function of the *electron transport chain* as it utilizes oxygen to make energy. It is interchangeable with mitochondrial combustion to make energy.

aging coefficient: Defined in minutes as a ratio of maximum exercise, using a standard format exercise test (Bruce), between predicted maximum peak exercise expected at age twenty-five and actual exercise performance. As an example, if the maximum amount of exercise for individual X was ten minutes on the treadmill and the expected amount of exercise for individual X was twenty minutes at age twenty-five, the aging coefficient would be 0.5. Interpreted, individual X has aged 50 percent from his or her optimal exercise baseline, implying a significant decline of skeletal-muscle tone and suggesting progressive inflammatory risk progression.

albumin: A protein in the blood, manufactured by the liver, that is critical to numerous cellular functions as it becomes a transporter protein and facilitates homeostasis of delicate pressure gradients between membranes.

aldehyde dehydrogenase: A family of nineteen different enzymes, with activity in liver, kidney, and brain cells, that oxidize acetaldehydes. In this book, it is referenced in *beta-oxidation* of *fatty acids*.

allopathic: A term to describe medical expertise utilizing government-approved medications, tests, and procedures to diagnose and treat medical conditions. These practitioners are often MDs (*medical doctors*) or DOs (*doctors of osteopathy*), but can also be FNPs (*family nurse practitioners*), and are strictly licensed and regulated. Other practitioners include *naturopaths* (NPs) and *homeopaths*. These healers often utilize alternative treatments that are often complementary to traditional treatments. Their emphasis is more preventative and involves changes in diet and living environment. They often use supplements, music, meditation, massage, and other accents to support *holistic* treatment strategies.

alpha-lipoic acid (ALA): A short-chain omega-3 fatty acid utilized in mitochondrial energy combustion and as a free-radical scavenger. It works in combination with vitamins C and E to prevent free-radical chain reactions.

alveoli: Lung epithelial cells at the very end of the pulmonary bronchial tree that specialize in oxygen and carbon dioxide gas exchange.

amino acids: Ubiquitous molecules that are the building blocks for production of proteins and enzymes.

amyloid: A mix of collagen and protein molecules that can accumulate in the interstitial space of any deteriorating end organ but is commonly found in compromised brain, liver, and kidney cells. Amyloid production can arise from *glial astrocyte cells* in the brain and is typically secreted when there is compromised capillary-cell function related to reductions in blood flow and increased inflammation in the interstitial space of the brain related to the risk for *hypoxic-ischemic events*. Because of chronically reduced blood flow, and hence oxygen delivery, it is postulated that amyloid, and its cousin *tau,* are types of scar tissue that form in the interstitial space, replacing normal brain cells as they atrophy and die from lack of oxygen (chronic hypoxia-ischemia). Buildup of amyloid and tau is correlated with progressive *dementia.*

anaerobic exercise: See aerobic exercise.

anemia: Occurs when there is a decrease in red blood cell volumes in the blood. It is often measured by blood *hematocrit* and *hemoglobin* levels. Anemia can be caused by blood loss (iron deficiency), diminished B_{12} (*cyanocobalamin*) and B_9 (*folate/folic acid*) levels, or many different chronic inflammatory conditions that suppress red blood cell production.

aneurysm: A dangerous ballooning dilatation of the walls of large arteries, which can eventually lead to rupture of the wall if not repaired. Aneurysms commonly occur in the *aorta* and are related to vascular

209

inflammatory risks, particularly cigarette smoking. There can also be an inherited predisposition to aneurysm formation.

angina pectoris: Refers to chest, arm, neck, or back pains, excessive fatigue or shortness of breath associated with strenuous activity or excessive stress, indicative of *coronary artery disease* (critical large-vessel narrowing of heart arteries). Coronary artery disease (CAD) is linked to family genetics and vascular inflammatory risks, particularly elevated blood sugars, LDL cholesterol, hypertension, and cigarette smoking. The development of angina pectoris implies the need for urgency in developing a treatment strategy to prevent a heart attack or sudden death.

angioedema: Generalized swelling, which can be life threatening if involving the tongue and neck, often related to a drug allergy, bee sting, or insect bite.

angiotensin II: A molecule that causes the smooth muscles surrounding *endothelial cells* of the vascular tree (other than capillary cells, which do not have surrounding smooth muscle) to contract, thereby narrowing their *lumens* and increasing blood pressure. If sustained, blood pressures and *shear stress* increase. Angiotensin II blood levels increase with age and aggregate vascular inflammatory risks. Its production requires collaboration of liver, kidney, and lung cells.

angiotensin converting enzyme inhibitors (ACEs): Drugs that block angiotensin II production, thereby reversing the proinflammatory effects of sustained increases in blood pressure, shear stress, and subsequent end-organ damage.

angiotensin receptor blockers (ARBs): Drugs that block angiotensin II receptors on membrane surfaces, thereby reversing the proinflammatory effects of sustained increases in blood pressure, shear stress, and subsequent end-organ damage. Using an ARB with an ACE inhibitor is *not* additive in this effect.

anion: A negatively charged ion, often masked as a free radical. (Compare with **cation**.)

antihypertensives: Medications that lower blood pressure. Commonly prescribed agents include ACEs, ARBs, diuretics, beta-blockers, and calcium channel blockers.

antioxidants: Vitamins, enzymes, and other molecules that neutralize *free radicals* to mitigate their proinflammatory effects. Chronic inflammation and age bias decrease in antioxidant levels in capillary and end-organ cells, thereby increasing the risk for free-radical damage to membranes and DNA. Examples of antioxidants are *vitamins C* and *E*, *glutathione, alpha-lipoic acid* (ALA), and superoxide dismutase.

anxiolytics: A group of medications that reduce anxiety. Most of these medications are addictive when used regularly.

aorta: The largest artery in the body. It originates at the aortic valve of the heart and subsequently branches off into numerous arteries that feed all the major end organs of the body.

apoptosis: A synonym for cell or organelle death (used in clinical settings).

arginine: Along with *citrulline,* this is a precursor to nitric oxide production.

arterial tree: The entire vasculature that supports oxygen, nutrient, and immune-arsenal delivery to the capillary infrastructure of all end organs.

astaxanthin: A potent fat-soluble antioxidant (electron donor) that may extend life expectancy and is found in plants and fish. It gives fresh salmon its dark-pink hue.

astrocytes: Specialized glial connective tissue cells that compose the *blood-brain barrier.*

autoimmune disease: An immune derangement in which an immune protein attaches to a normal cellular protein, creating a proinflammatory complex that can plume additional inflammation in the interstitial space of end organs. Autoimmune complexes always increase inflammation and adversely impact function to affected end organs.

autophagy: Occurs when a cell or organelle commits suicide. Capillary-cell mitochondria execute autophagy by forming a large pore (hole) and merging into it. When they do, they are disassembled.

basal energy: The amount of energy that a cell utilizes to maintain everyday function. At the capillary level, it usually does not include sudden surges of energy required by outer membranes to activate active transport of inflammatory mediators.

basement membrane: For the purposes of this book, this represents a specialized abluminal outer membrane of endothelial and capillary cells that serves the special needs of smooth-muscle cells or the end organ they serve.

beta-blockers: A class, or family, of medicines that lower blood pressure and protect heart function.

beta-oxidation: A process that occurs in the *mitochondrial matrix* to metabolize *fatty acids* to *acetyl CoA*, which can then enter the *Krebs cycle* or be utilized for *protein synthesis* or *mitochondrial replication.*

blood-brain barrier: A protective barrier to the brain and spinal cord, composed of *capillary cells, astrocytes,* and *pericytes.* It provides the brain with *cerebrospinal fluid* (CSF), a clear, colorless bath of oxygen, nutrients, and electrolytes.

body mass index (BMI): A method of defining obesity and malnutrition. BMIs greater than 30 are defined as obese and greater than 35 as morbidly obese. In nonathletes, BMIs less than 18 are considered malnourished.

bradykinin: An inflammatory mediator that has predominantly proinflammatory effects.

brain fog: A syndrome caused from combinations of inflammatory factors that diminish *cognition,* the capacity to think coherently, problem solve, remember, and learn.

bronchi/bronchial tree: A group of bifurcating cartilage-based tubes in the lung, beginning at the trachea and culminating in breathing sacs of gas exchange known as *alveoli.*

calcium: A cation mineral stored in the *mitochondrial matrix* and adjacent *smooth endoplasmic reticulum* of capillary cells. When released, calcium facilitates increased capillary-cell outer-membrane permeability to inflammatory mediators by reducing outer-membrane voltage gradients and inducing actin-myosin fibril contraction, thereby opening the gap-junction orifice between capillary cells.

calcium channel blockers: A family of medicines that lower blood pressure by blocking smooth-muscle calcium ion channels in large arteries, thereby relaxing smooth-muscle cells that surround large vessel arteries. This relaxation causes lumen diameters to increase, which then lowers resistance to flow through them, thereby lowering blood pressure.

calcium ion flux: The movement of calcium ions into and out of mitochondria and *smooth endoplasmic reticulum* to capillary-cell outer membranes to activate enzymes and voltage gradients that increase or decrease permeability.

capillary cells: A specialized *endothelial cell* that lacks a smooth-muscle coat and specializes in protecting their respective end organ's interstitial space from inflammatory influences and supporting end-organ function.

carbon monoxide: A colorless, odorless but very dangerous gas by-product of cigarette smoke. Besides being a carcinogen, carbon monoxide binds to *hemoglobin* to limit its capacity to transport and exchange oxygen by diffusion through capillary cells.

carcinogens: Chemicals, gases, or free radicals that are known to cause cancer.

carnitine palmitoyltransferase (CPT-1): A family of at least three enzymes that can convert certain *fatty acids* in the cytoplasm to acyl carnitines, which allows them to be transported into the mitochondria and through *beta-oxidation* to make acetyl CoA. CPT-1 deficiency causes *hypoglycemia* and *brain nerve-cell damage.*

carotid artery: A major artery of the arterial tree that bifurcates into the internal and external carotid arteries, which then supply the brain with blood, oxygen, and nutrients. The two carotid arteries flow on each side of the neck and become vulnerable to plaque development where they bifurcate, as a result of aggregates of increased shear stress and other vascular inflammatory free radicals.

cation: A positively charged ion, such as hydrogen (protons) or heavy metals or salt (calcium, sodium, potassium, magnesium, iron, selenium, copper, manganese, zinc). (Compare with **anion**.) Cations are important in establishing membrane voltage gradients and pumps, as transporters, in facilitating electron transfer, and as cofactors in metabolism, protein synthesis, and replication. They also can act as *antioxidants* or can become *free radicals.*

cellulitis: Inflammation/infection of the skin that includes the epidermis, dermis, and at times, the adjacent subcutaneous fat.

cerebrospinal fluid (CSF): The clear, colorless, odorless bath of fluid that is produced by a specialized group of capillary cells in the *choroid plexus* and facilitated by specific *blood-brain barrier* exchanges throughout the capillary cell network of the brain and spinal cord.

choroid plexus: A specialized group of capillary cells deep in the brain (lateral ventricles) that produces *cerebrospinal fluid* (CSF).

chromosomes: These are found in the nucleus or mitochondria and carry DNA, which codes for the replication of all the capillary- and endothelial-cell outer-membrane receptor proteins, organelles, and infrastructure of the cell. Each cell's nucleus has twenty-three pairs of chromosomes.

chronic obstructive pulmonary disease (COPD): Usually the outcome of chronic inflammation of lung tissue, resulting in diminished capacity to take deep breaths and blow air out quickly. COPD can be measured by pulmonary function testing. It is graded as mild, moderate, or severe, and often has reactive (asthma), restrictive, and obstructive components.

cirrhosis: Occurs when liver cells (*hepatocytes*) are exposed to chronic inflammatory processes in their interstitial space, usually from chronic alcohol exposure. The space becomes overrun with fibrous scar tissue, increasing risks for cancer and infection, decreasing hepatocyte and liver function, and increasing fatigue, pain, and aging.

cis fat: A fat that can have anti-inflammatory properties. Cis fats, particularly vegetable oils, when utilized for cooking or baking, may reconfigure to *trans fats*, which are very proinflammatory. Trans fats may assemble on capillary- and endothelial-cell outer membranes to cause increases in permeability to inflammatory mediators. Saturated or monounsaturated oils are more stable when heated and are less likely to convert to trans fats.

citrulline: A precursor to nitric oxide combustion.

clotting factors: Circulating molecules produced in the liver that, when activated by another clotting factor, *thrombin,* cascade clot formation. As proinflammatory mediators and chronic inflammation increase in the interstitial space of end organs or larger vessels in the endothelium, pro-clotting biases increase.

clotting function: Laboratory measurements that determine the quality and quantity of clot formation.

coenzyme Q_{10} (CoQ$_{10}$): Also called *ubiquinone* (UQ), this is a critical cofactor in *electron transport* of the *cytochrome system* of the *mitochondrial inner membrane.* It also acts as a *free-radical scavenger* or *antioxidant.* In this sense, CoQ$_{10}$ facilitates both energy combustion and removal of the toxic free-radical exhaust the combustion creates. CoQ$_{10}$ levels decreases with age, and its production is blocked by *statins.*

collateral circulation: Accessory or duplicate blood flow of an artery to an end organ. This becomes critically important when oxygen-sensitive end organs, such as the brain or heart, have arteries blocked from *obstructive plaque* that prevents blood flow. Having collateral circulation from a different blood vessel supplying the same area of the brain or heart often saves the tissue from *hypoxic* injury.

complement system: A family of twenty different proteins that are made in the liver and circulate in the blood. They are utilized as part of the immune-arsenal response of *white blood cells, cytokines,* and *immunoglobulins* to isolate and eliminate an inflammatory breach.

complex carbohydrates (polysaccharides): Structures with multiple carbon rings and branched chains of carbons, they are larger and more complex than smaller carbohydrates. Their molecular complexity is a key to their health benefits, as they are more difficult to break down into simple sugars; therefore, they are beneficial to metabolism, as they trickle rather than tsunami into liver *hepatocytes,* as simple sugars often do. Additionally, complex carbohydrate metabolism (as compared to that of simple sugars) is linked to ingestion of more plants fiber, improved intestinal microbiome constituency, increased absorption of vitamins and antioxidants, and reduced risk for diabetes, elevated LDL cholesterol, or hypertension.

computerized tomography (CT): A type of advanced two- and three-dimensional imaging.

coronary artery disease (CAD): The development of plaque in the large arterial vessels that supply heart muscle. CAD is caused by vascular inflammatory free-radical seeding and inflammatory-mediator pluming over an extended period of time, and can lead to chest pains (*angina pectoris*), heart attacks, arrhythmias, congestive heart failure, and sudden death.

coronary calcium scores (CCS): An imaging test that measures the volume of calcium that has deposited in coronary arteries. The implication is that larger volumes are linked to greater risk of heart attacks. CCS may also be important in determining a similar risk to brain vascular events and subsequent dementia.

cortisol: A stress hormone made in the adrenal glands that becomes a vascular inflammatory mediator when produced in excess.

covalent ions: A chemical bond that involves the sharing of two electrons. This type of bond is considered more stable than a single-electron bond and therefore not as risky to become an oxidized *free radical. Antioxidants* can utilize covalent bonding to prevent free-radical chain reactions.

critical large-vessel plaque: Also known as *large-vessel symptomatic plaque,* this occurs when plaque in large vessels has increased in size, usually to *occlude* 70 percent or more of the *lumen* of the vessel. When this occurs in highly oxygen-dependent end organs (heart, brain), symptoms such as chest pains or ministrokes (TIAs) emerge. If left untreated, this plaque leads to dangerous risks for heart failure and dementia.

crustaceans: Usually referred to as a krill, shrimp, crab, lobster, or barnacle. Crustaceans often have a dark-orange shell and have been linked to substances (*astaxanthin, omega-3 oils*) that have *antioxidant* and antiaging properties. As crustaceans get older, many of them do not appear to demonstrate typical characteristics of aging.

cyclic AMP (cAMP-cyclic adenosine monophosphate): Activated through the conversion of ATP, cAMP becomes one of several feedback-loop switches that affect capillary-cell outer-membrane permeability to inflammatory mediators, as well as affecting enzymes such as PKA (*protein kinase A*), which modulates *sugars* and *fatty acids* across membrane surfaces.

cysteine: An *amino acid* that is a precursor to *glutathione,* a potent all-purpose *antioxidant* in all cells. When ingested as *N-acetyl cysteine* (NAC), it is better absorbed. With aging or chronic inflammation, cysteine often gets converted to *homocysteine,* which, in contrast to glutathione, is a very sticky, proinflammatory seeding molecule that plumes vascular inflammatory mediators into interstitial spaces of end organs and is linked to *dementia.*

cytochrome: A group of five complexes on the *mitochondrial inner membrane* that pass electrons through a series of chemical reactions to eventually result in the production of large volumes of ATP. The cytochrome system is the key piece to mitochondrial energy combustion as well as to maintaining the *inner-membrane voltage gradient.*

cytokines: A family of *pleotropic* proteins that act as pro- or anti-inflammatory mediators. They are produced by endothelial cells, including capillary cells, as well as various white blood cells, liver, end-organ, and mesenchymal cells.

cytoplasm: Refers to the inside substance of any cell and is where the nucleus, mitochondria, and other organelles reside.

dementia: Cognitive decline that affects capacity to remember, learn, adapt, problem solve, move, and balance. It is also linked to decreased hearing, vision, and sense of smell. Dementia is usually screened by simple testing known as the MMSE (*mini mental status exam*) and confirmed by imaging studies and other tests. It is often associated with movement disorders, such as *Parkinson's disease*. Dementia increases dramatically with age and accumulating vascular inflammatory free radicals tied to sleep deprivation, cigarette smoking, diabetes, sugar intake, hypertension, increased LDL cholesterol, obesity, and immobility. It is almost universally linked to *cerebral atrophy* (loss of brain volume) evident on imaging studies as well as to buildup of *amyloid* and *tau* plaques.

diabetes mellitus: A fasting blood sugar (no food after midnight) of 126 mg/dL or higher, coupled with a *hemoglobin A1C* of 6.5 or higher. *Prediabetes* (*insulin resistance*) is defined as a fasting blood sugar of 101–125 mg/dL and a hemoglobin A1C of 5.7–6.4. Vascular inflammatory risk escalates as hemoglobin A1C increases above 5.6.

diffusion: The movement of gases or molecules across membranes without the need for energy.

digital thermal monitoring (DTM): A novel method of measuring capillary-cell health as depicted by the rate and volume of nitric oxide production after creating skeletal-muscle *hypoxia* by using an arm cuff. The faster and more robust the response after release of the blood pressure cuff (based on a thermal return to a finger monitor), the better the overall health of the capillary cell. The response becomes an indirect indicator of capillary cell mitochondrial volumes.

disaccharides: Simple sugars that are abundant in Western diets, are hidden constituents in many processed foods, and are vascular inflammatory. A common misconception is that simple sugars must taste sweet. This is only true for sucrose and fructose. Also known as "empty calories," they are linked to an inferior intestinal microbiome, fatty liver, diabetes, metabolic syndrome, obesity, increases in LDL cholesterol, and hypertension. (See also **monosaccharides** and **trisaccharides**.)

DNA: Genetic material composed of sequenced nucleic acids on chromosomes that code for protein synthesis. Nuclear chromosomal DNA is covered with a *telomere cap* for protection, whereas *mitochondrial DNA* is not. With DNA damage from free radicals, protein synthesis becomes defective.

docosahexaenoic acid (DHA): An essential long-chain fatty acid made from its precursor, *eicosapentaenoic acid* (EPA). DHA is found in high concentrations in salmon and tuna and has extensive vascular anti-inflammatory properties. With age, chronic illness, and aggregate vascular risks, blood levels decline. (See also **eicosapentaenoic acid**.)

drug addiction: Occurs when certain drugs, prescription or otherwise (opioids, alcohol, methamphetamines, barbiturates, anxiolytics, sleeping pills), ingested over time result in *drug tolerance* (less effective than intended effect), as well as physical and psychological dependency. Over time, drug requirements usually increase, and withdrawal of the drug can produce serious side effects, including seizures and even death. These substances eventually become vascular inflammatory.

drug tolerance: Occurs when the desired effect(s) of a drug become less effective over time. This is often mitigated by increasing the dose, which then accelerates side effects.

echocardiogram/echocardiography: A noninvasive method of looking at the structure and function of the heart in two and three dimensions.

edema: Swelling of the skin and subcutaneous tissues, often in dependent areas like the legs and feet.

eicosapentaenoic acid (EPA): An essential long-chain fatty acid with anti-inflammatory properties. It lowers serum triglyceride levels and can be converted in most cells to DHA, which is considered to have even more vascular anti-inflammatory properties. (See also **docosahexaenoic acid.**)

electrolytes: A family of common molecules that include sodium, potassium, chloride, and bicarbonate. Together, they facilitate *membrane voltage gradients,* serve as buffers, and promote expansion or contraction of water volumes in a cell.

electromechanical gradient (EM gradient): A variable but unique electrical gradient on most membrane surfaces that is often mediated by a sodium/potassium pump and blocked (decreased membrane gradient) by calcium ions. When voltage gradients decrease on outer membranes, permeability of molecules through them increases. Capillary cells of the *blood-brain barrier* have a potent outer membrane EM gradient, as does the capillary-cell *mitochondrial inner membrane.* This membrane gradient helps protect imbalances of hydrogen ions in the *mitochondrial intermembrane space* and calcium ions in the *mitochondrial matrix.* Maintaining the gradient is vital to the mitochondrial pendulum swing of combustion, which in turn regulates homeostasis of *heme production, calcium storage and release, ATP/ADP ratios, energy and nitric oxide production,* and *ROS balance and feedback loops* to other membranes and organelles.

electron transport chain (ETC): The series of protein electron carriers in the five-chamber *cytochrome complex* on the *inner membrane of* *mitochondria* that eventually cause the *phosphorylation* of ADP to ATP, which is the basic energy unit of all cells. The ETC plays a major role in also maintaining the *electromechanical gradient* between the *mitochondrial intermembrane space* and *matrix*.

empty calories: A term used to describe highly processed, predominantly simple-carbohydrate snack foods in which most of the vitamin and mineral content has been leached out by processing. The term has been extended to include most colas and fruit juices.

end organs: The organs that capillary cells facilitate. End organs include brain, heart, skeletal muscle, lungs, kidneys, liver, sex organs, adrenal glands, eyes, ears, nose, peripheral nerves, and teeth, among others. For arterial endothelial cells, the end organ is the *smooth-muscle cells* that surround them and cause their *lumens* to relax or constrict, thereby increasing or decreasing resistance and blood pressures through them.

endocytosis: An energy transport mechanism in which a molecule is engulfed (swallowed), typically at an outer membrane, encapsulated into a vesicle, transported through the cell, and then released into the interstitial space on the opposite (*abluminal*) side of the capillary cell.

endoplasmic reticulum (ER): Can be smooth or rough. *Rough ER* contains *ribosomes* and is involved in the mechanics of *protein synthesis*. The *smooth ER* is intimately tied to mitochondria in the capillary cell and serves as an additional reservoir for *calcium ion storage*. It also is involved in the breakdown and recycling of intermediates to *heme*.

endothelial cells: The innermost lining of cells of the vascular system that are exposed to blood constituents. They also include vein and lymph vessels.

endothelin: A molecule that can be produced by *endothelial cells*, causing smooth muscle to contract, decreasing lumen diameter, and increasing blood pressures through arterial vessels.

endothelium: All the cells that line the vascular tree (also known as *endothelial cells*). *Capillary cells* are specialized endothelial cells that have adapted their outer membranes to facilitate end-organ function.

energy substrate: *Pyruvate* (from *glucose* and *glycogen*), *fatty acids* (from *glycerol*), and *ketone bodies* (from fatty acids). In the mitochondria, all energy substrate goes to *acetyl CoA*, which can be catabolized in the *Krebs cycle* for subsequent energy production, or shunted away from the Krebs cycle and toward cytoplasmic ribosomes and rough endoplasmic reticulum for *protein synthesis* and *mitochondrial replication*.

enterohepatic circulation: In this context, an older term that refers to portal vein blood that transfers nutrients from the microbiome and intestinal epithelial cells, where it admixes with portal arterial blood in the *liver sinusoid* to eventually be introduced to liver *hepatocytes* through a very porous capillary cell.

enzymes: Molecules that catalyze reactions. That is, enzyme reactions are part of a check-and-balance feedback-loop system. Free radicals, on the other hand, cause reactions to occur that are not caused from enzymes and are generally not a part of a check-and-balance feedback-loop system. Free radicals are also generally proinflammatory, whereas enzyme reactions can increase or decrease inflammation based on feedback loops activated.

epithelium/epithelial cells: Specialized cells that compose all end organs.

essential vitamins and minerals: Constituents that must be ingested for the body to utilize them. They cannot be manufactured within the human body.

estrogen: Female hormone that, along with progesterone, is made in the ovary. Levels fluctuate based on the timing of the menstrual cycle.

With menopause, levels decrease substantially and are associated with hot flashes, insomnia, depression, weight gain, and dry skin.

exocytosis: Process by which molecules are transported in capillary or endothelial cells from the cell's abluminal side to its luminal side utilizing vesicles and active-transport mechanics.

ezetimibe: Decreases LDL cholesterol by interfering with its absorption through the intestines.

FAD/FADH: *Flavin adenine dinucleotide* (FAD) and *reduced flavin adenine dinucleotide* (FADH) are found in high concentrations in the *mitochondrial matrix* and serve to deposit hydrogen into the *cytochrome system* for purposes of *electron transport.*

fatty acids: Fat molecules that are broken down in mitochondria through *beta-oxidation* to make *acetyl CoA.* They compete with *pyruvate* (glucose), and when used, it is thought that they produce more ROS (*free-radical exhaust*) than pyruvate when producing acetyl CoA.

feedback loop: A signaling process where a message chain-reacts in the cell. As an example, the presence of inflammatory mediators in the interstitial space of an end organ increases capillary-cell outer-membrane permeability, which produces feedback loops that chain-react more permeability and subsequent movement of more inflammatory mediators into the interstitial space for removal of inflammatory seeds. This process requires energy, so a feedback loop is made with mitochondria to increase energy combustion to make more ATP to facilitate active-transport processes.

fenestrae: Also called *fenestrations*, these are capillary-cell outer-membrane *pores*. Fenestrae come in different sizes and volumes within a given capillary cell, and most have diaphragms that further filter contents through them. When capillary-cell outer membranes *pseudocapillarize*, pore diversity and volume decrease, which limits capillary cell–sequenced immune responses to inflammation. Even so, with pseudocapillarization, net permeability through outer membranes of inflammatory mediators actually increases.

fibromyalgia: More common in women, this condition involves diffuse muscle pain involving multiple symmetric muscles in the shoulders, torso, and legs. It is highly correlated with a previous history of physical trauma, sustained stress, and chronic insomnia. It is often mistaken for *chronic fatigue syndrome* (also known as SEID [*systemic exertion intolerance disease*]). Treatment involves stress reduction, symptomatic pain management, and efforts to reduce sleep deprivation. It is thought that reducing vascular inflammatory free radicals may also improve fibromyalgia.

free radicals: Negatively or positively charged molecules with exposed electrons that can attach to surface membranes or DNA to alter their function and create plumes of additional inflammation. Free-radical reactions are in contrast to *enzyme reactions,* which are linked to cross-checks and feedback loops to increase or decrease their activity. Free radicals may occur from vascular inflammatory mediators (e.g., LDL cholesterol, tobacco toxins, and AGEs) or because of combustion exhaust from mitochondria (superoxide and hydrogen peroxide from energy combustion, or hydroxynitrite from nitric oxide exhaust).

free-radical scavengers: Another name for *antioxidants* that neutralize (or reduce) free radicals.

gap junction: The space between cells. Between capillary cells, the gap junction can be tight when tight borders are required (*blood-brain barrier*) to keep blood constituents away from the end organ, or loose, such as in the *liver sinusoid*. With inflammation in the interstitial space, the gap-junction orifice widens to accommodate more permeability and movement of *inflammatory mediators* into the interstitial space to plume the inflammatory response.

gastroesophageal reflux disease (GERD): Also referred to as *symptomatic reflux of acid* (heartburn) from the stomach into the esophagus.

gene silencing: Occurs when free radicals cross-link DNA to "silence" their intended purpose.

genomics: The genetic makeup of the cell. It involves the specific sequencing of *chromosomal DNA*, which forms the blueprint for protein synthesis and cell function. The cell's genomics are found in its nucleus and mitochondria.

glial cells: Connective-tissue cells in the brain and spinal cord, including oligodendrocytes, ependymal cells, and astrocytes. Knowledge of their functional importance and interaction with nerve cells is expanding greatly. *Astrocytes,* along with *pericytes* and *capillary cells,* compose the *blood-brain barrier.* Under duress that is often related to chronic inflammation from vascular inflammatory free radicals and subsequent hypoxemia, the astrocytes secrete a sticky *amyloid* coat on adjacent nerve cells, which correlates with their underperformance and atrophy.

glomerulonephritis: A nonspecific term signifying inflammation in the interstitial space between capillary and podocyte cells, which is adversely affecting filtration. The urine typically has a complement of protein, red blood cells, and epithelial-cell casts, reflecting an active sediment or *slough* from chronic glomerular inflammation.

glomerulus: The capsular-like structure or first part of the kidney *nephron* unit, where initial filtering of blood plasma occurs to make *ultrafiltrate.*

gluconeogenesis: The reverse of *glycolysis,* where energy is utilized to convert pyruvate back to glucose. Gluconeogenesis can be linked to *insulin resistance* and persistently increases in cells when there is abundant energy substrate, excessive caloric intake, or underutilization of energy substrate from inactivity. It is observed in advanced age, with inactivity, and with obesity. Gluconeogenesis is vascular proinflammatory and predisposes to *adult-onset diabetes*.

glucose: A six-carbon simple sugar (*monosaccharide*) that is typically reduced in the cytoplasm (*glycolysis*) and mitochondria of cells to a three-carbon molecule known as *pyruvate*. Pyruvate competes with *fatty acids* in the *mitochondrial matrix* as a substrate to make *acetyl CoA*. Other simple sugars include fructose, sucrose (table sugar), galactose, lactose, maltose, sorbitol, and alcohol sugars. Chronic and persistent increases in blood sugar (*diabetes*) are highly vascular inflammatory, accelerate aging, increase AGEs, and are considered a major vascular inflammatory–mediator risk.

glutathione: A potent all-purpose *antioxidant* (free-radical scavenger) found in all cells and produced from *cysteine*. Levels decrease with age and chronic interstitial-space inflammation.

glycation: Implies the dangerous predisposition of glucose becoming a free radical (AGE), binding to a membrane protein, without the aid of an enzyme, to cause membrane disruption.

glycemic index: An index based on how much the food increases blood sugar. Foods high on the glycemic index increase blood sugars quickly and to higher levels. It must be understood that all simple sugars can do this; therefore, lactose in bread, although not sweet, has a very high glycemic index. Potatoes, although not sweet, also have a very high glycemic index.

glycerol storage: How fat is stored in *adipose* tissue (fat cells).

glycocalyx: A *glycoprotein* (protein with glucose and carbohydrate) that serves as a coat, or extra barrier of protection, to the continuous outer-membrane luminal side of the capillary cell. With chronic inflammation, the glycocalyx decreases in thickness or disappears entirely. The loss of the glycocalyx connotes *pseudocapillarization* and biases capillary-cell outer membranes to increase permeability to inflammatory mediators.

glycogen: The carbohydrate storage product in the liver.

glycolysis: The anaerobic process in the cytoplasm in which *glucose* is converted to *pyruvate*, which is then utilized as a substrate in the *mitochondrial matrix* to make *acetyl CoA*.

guanosine diphosphate (GDP): Can be phosphorylated to *guanosine triphosphate* (GTP), utilizing oxygen and phosphorus is a similar fashion of ADP to ATP. The resultant GTP can be used in the cell as an alternative energy source for specific functions by releasing phosphorus to form GDP.

hematocrit: A measurement of *red blood cell* volume in the blood plasma.

heme synthesis: Occurs in the *mitochondrial matrix*, where iron is encircled with a crown of carbons and then utilized as heme in the *cytochrome system* to pass electrons.

hemoglobin: A molecule carried by all *red blood cells*, its purpose is to transport and exchange oxygen by diffusion through capillary cells.

hemoglobin A1C (HbA1C): A sensitive *blood plasma* marker indicative of how much inflammation is present as a result of elevated blood sugars. Higher numbers imply inadequate blood sugar management and carry an increased risk for vascular inflammatory consequences. Values of 5.6 or less are normal. Medications are required for levels greater than 7.

hepatic portal blood/circulation: Used in this book to indicate nutrient-rich blood being transported from the microbiome-intestinal portal vein to the liver sinusoids, where it is unloaded to liver *hepatocytes* for subsequent manufacturing and distribution.

hepatocytes: Liver parenchymal cells.

high-density lipoprotein (HDL) cholesterol: Also known as "good" cholesterol, this is a vascular inflammatory risk factor when blood levels fall below 40 mg/dL. Although raising HDL cholesterol above 40 mg/dL has merit, increasing HDL further with medications, such as *niacin,* does not improve vascular risk. The number-one priority in lipid management is to decrease LDL cholesterol levels below 100 mg/dL.

highly sensitive C-reactive protein (HS-CRP): An excellent marker of vascular inflammation, but it can be elevated by other causes of inflammation, such as cancer, infection, and autoimmune disease.

histamine: A well-known vascular inflammatory mediator, histamine plumes inflammation within the interstitial space.

HMG-CoA reductase inhibitors: Also known as *statins,* these medications lower LDL cholesterol by blocking its production in the liver. (Compare with **statins.**)

homeostasis: The capacity of all the cells and organs of the human organism to maintain optimal function based on an internal system of checks and balances and feedback loops.

homocysteine: An abnormally sticky molecule that acts as a *free-radical seed* and globs onto membranes to plume inflammation and disrupt their function. It is linked to *dementia* and to *ineffective metabolism of cofactors*—folate, pyridoxine, and cyanocobalamin—of cysteine.

hydrogen: For the purposes of this book, *hydrogen* refers to positively charged ions (also known as protons) that facilitate *mitochondrial matrix inner-membrane gradients* and are utilized by the fifth *cytochrome* in combination with ADP, ATP synthetase, phosphorus, and oxygen to make energy (ATP). When inner-membrane proteins become defective, hydrogen leaks back into the matrix, thereby weakening the inner-membrane voltage gradient.

hydroxyl nitrite: A type of toxic free-radical exhaust from mitochondrial nitric oxide combustion.

hypertension: Persistent elevation in blood pressure greater than 140/90 mm/Hg. Borderline hypertension are readings of 121–139/85–90 mm/Hg, taken by a cuff wrapped around the biceps and triceps muscles of the arm.

hypoglycemia: Defined as blood sugars dropping below 70 mg/dL. Similar symptoms can occur to mimic hypoglycemia in patients with a rapid descent in blood sugars that may not drop below 100 mg/dL.

hypothalamus: Structure in the brain near the pituitary gland. It releases various hormones that regulate growth, metabolism, and sex.

hypoxia: The state that results when arterial blood oxygen levels diminish to a point that adversely affects end-organ function. Heart and brain function are very sensitive to sustained reductions in oxygen levels.

immune arsenal: Second-line, inside-out inflammatory mediators composed of families of white blood cells, cytokines, complement, immunoglobulins, and platelets that respond to first-line, often outside-in inflammatory mediator risks or seeds that plume an inflammatory response to eliminate inflammatory breach. When unsuccessful, chronic inflammation within the interstitial space results.

immune mediators: Similar to the immune arsenal.

immune support: Similar to and interchangeable with immune arsenal and mediators.

immune surveillance: It is the function of capillary-cell outer membranes to modulate an effective, sequenced immune response consisting of inflammatory mediators to eliminate interstitial-space inflammatory breach and maintain interstitial-space hygiene. Doing so supports improved end-organ function and requires an effective back-and-forth capillary-cell outer-membrane permeability pivot and mitochondrial combustion pendulum swing dance.

immune system: Many of these constituents originate from lymph tissue, spleen, bone marrow, and liver, but many cytokines are growth factors produced locally by endothelial, mesenchymal, and end-organ cells. All are integrated by capillary-cell outer membranes to form an effective response to eliminate inflammatory interstitial-space breach. (See also **immune arsenal** and **immune mediators**.)

immunoglobulin: Large, bulky proteins that are programmed to attach to foreign protein receptors to form an antigen-antibody complex that is then identified and removed.

inflammatory mediators: May cause or be the effect of an immune response. First-line inflammatory mediators (vascular inflammatory free radicals) often initiate inflammation by seeding the end organ's interstitial space and endothelial- and capillary-cell basement membranes. They subsequently create an immune arsenal response commensurate with their seeding, which plumes additional inflammation in attempts to remove the inflammatory breach. (See **immune arsenal**.)

insomnia: Refers to the decreased capacity to fall and stay asleep, and also to continuous sleep that is consistently less than seven hours. Insomnia becomes a major cause of sleep deprivation. Its multiple causes, which become more common in middle age, must be ferreted out and treated.

insulin resistance: With increasing age, obesity, eating processed foods with high glycemic indexes, immobility, sarcopenia, and genetic predisposition, fasting blood sugars increase to greater than 100 mg/dL, and hemoglobin A1C increases to 5.7–6.4. Insulin resistance is another name for *prediabetes* and infers the beginning of vascular inflammatory risks from risking blood sugars.

interstitial space: The space between the capillary and end-organ cell. It is where cellular business is conducted, involving the exchanges of oxygen, nutrients, waste, and other blood plasma constituents between the blood and end organ.

ions: These are charged molecules (they can be negatively or positively charged). When ions are exposed because of the configuration of the molecule, they can facilitate enzymatic reactions; in a more sinister fashion, they can act as free radicals, attaching to and damaging membranes and DNA.

ischemia: Describes what can happen to an end organ when there is insufficient blood flow and/or lack of oxygen to support function. Ischemia can lead to hypoxic-ischemic events in oxygen-sensitive end organs. Such events include *myocardial infarction* (heart) and *TIAs/ strokes* (brain) that lead to congestive heart failure and dementia.

ketones: Produced from fatty acids in the liver as a result of very low-calorie diets or starvation.

ketosis: A result of a buildup of ketones in the bloodstream. Ketosis can be dangerous in *type 1 diabetes* (insulin-dependent diabetes), where ketosis can decrease blood pH, potentially leading to death if not urgently treated.

Krebs cycle: Takes *acetyl CoA* and metabolizes it to yield a small amount of ATP, but even more important, releases hydrogen ions, which can attach to FAD and NAD and then be mobilized to the *cytochrome* *system,* where they are deposited to facilitate the transport of electrons to eventually make large volumes of ATP.

Kupffer cells: Specialized *mesenchymal-helper cells* in the interstitial space of the *liver sinusoids* that assist the capillary cell in providing immune support to protect the space from unwanted invaders. This is a critical function of Kupffer cells because of the nature of capillary-cell function in this end organ. Since almost everything from the portal blood gets exposed to the liver cell, the Kupffer cell must be on guard to eliminate potential toxicities.

leaky gut syndrome: A process caused by malfunctioning of the *intestinal microbiome,* often as a result of a diet of *simple sugars* and *refined carbohydrates.* The altered microbiome cascades malabsorption of quality nutrient, which leaks back into feces while allowing more toxic constituents to be mobilized into the portal vein to be transported to the liver sinusoid. Leaky gut implies chronic interstitial-space inflammation between capillary and intestinal epithelial cells.

leptin: An important hormone released primarily by fat cells, it acts on the satiety center of the brain, within the *hypothalamus,* to decrease appetite. The effects of leptin may be negatively impacted by several mechanisms, leading to obesity. Intake of excessive sugar or sugar substitutes can block the effects of leptin on the hypothalamus. Increasing leptin production generally decreases appetite. The counterbalance to leptin is the hormone *ghrelin,* which is produced primarily in the stomach and increases appetite. Too much ghrelin or too little leptin can increase risk for obesity.

leukotrienes: A fat-soluble family of substances produced by *white blood cells* that becomes part of an *inflammatory plume* to eliminate foreign invaders, including particulates, viruses, bacteria, and cancer cells, from the interstitial space of end organs.

lipidemia: A condition where blood fat levels are elevated when tested in a fasting state (no food after midnight prior to testing). Lipid elevations can be *LDL cholesterol, triglycerides, lipoprotein (a),* and *non-HDL cholesterol.*

lipoprotein (a): Abbreviated *lipo(a),* this is a sticky, inflammatory, low-density cholesterol that globs onto membrane surfaces to trigger plumes of inflammation. It has an affinity for vascular membranes of high *shear stress,* such as carotid artery bifurcations and aortic valve cusps, but can also be linked to premature coronary artery disease. Treatment options to reduce lipo(a) are limited to the *niacins.*

low-density lipoprotein (LDL cholesterol): Also known as "bad" cholesterol, this is a highly vascular inflammatory cholesterol that, when small particle and oxidized, can attach as a *free radical* to cell membranes to plume an inflammatory response.

lumen: The space through which blood flows in an artery, vein, or lymph vessel.

magnesium: A critically important mineral that participates as a *cofactor* in many different cellular functions, as well as facilitating transport of ATP out of the *mitochondrial matrix* to the capillary-cell *outer membranes,* where it can be utilized for *active-transport processes.*

magnetic resonance imaging (MRI): An advanced type of imaging that can give very specific resolution in suspected disease. Utilizing MRI for purposes of screening for vascular inflammatory risks is expensive and not currently recommended.

manganese: An important mineral that is incorporated into the powerful antioxidant, *superoxide dismutase.*

manganese superoxide dismutase (MnSOD): Also known as SOD, this is a potent and specific *free-radical scavenger antioxidant* in the *mitochondrial matrix* that neutralizes superoxide, the primary toxic free radical of mitochondrial energy combustion. Both the production and levels of MnSOD decrease with age. Recently, levels of MnSOD have been increased in the mitochondrial matrix by attaching them to easily absorbable carrier proteins.

Mediterranean diet: Several studies have shown that a diet of fish, vegetables, monounsaturated oils, unprocessed food, and small amounts of red wine reduces all causes of death by up to 30 percent. Improvements from the diet directly correlate with reductions in vascular inflammatory free radicals and chronic inflammation.

mesenchymal cells: Also known as *mural* or *helper cells,* these specialized cells found in the interstitial space of end organs are designed to facilitate immune surveillance.

metabolic equivalent of task (MET): For the purposes of this book, MET is an estimate based on stress-testing protocols of maximum energy utilization. It can be used for several purposes, including the formulation of a safe exercise prescription. It can also be used as an *aging coefficient* and can serve as a proxy to estimate the degree of aging that has occurred in an individual in a given moment of time.

metabolic syndrome: A malignant, highly vascular inflammatory condition characterized by *diabetes, high LDL cholesterol, high blood pressure,* and *obesity.* It has become an epidemic in modern culture. It is linked to inactivity, snacking on highly processed sugary foods and drinks, insomnia, and night-shift work.

metformin: An oral hypoglycemic used to treat adult-onset diabetes, it has anti-inflammatory benefits based on its *pleotropic effect* on decreasing *gluconeogenesis,* thereby mimicking metabolic effects similar to exercise or low-calorie diets.

microbiome: The quality and quantity of bacteria in the intestines. The microbiome is improved by eating plant-based fiber and supplementing with probiotics.

mitochondria: Organelles found in all cells that have DNA and utilize oxygen to make energy and nitric oxide as part of a back-and-forth pendulum swing based on feedback-loop checks and balances from outer membranes and other signals. In capillary cells, mitochondrial combustion is based on feedback loops generated from outer-membrane permeability adjustments and hence can be described as *outer-membrane permeability pivoting* to cause *mitochondrial combustion pendulum swinging,* or the *capillary-cell dance.* An effective back-and-forth dance provides interstitial-space immune support, regulates blood flow and clotting dynamics, and rejuvenates the capillary-cell outer membranes to prepare for the next inflammatory free-radical onslaught. Mitochondria are composed of an *outer membrane, intermembrane space, inner membrane,* and *core matrix.* The inner membrane is defined by its powerful *electromechanical gradient* and five-chamber *cytochrome system* of *electron transport,* which is key to rapidly making substantial amounts of energy. *Mitochondrial chromosomal DNA* is also located in the matrix and is vulnerable to *free-radical oxidation* because of its proximity to oxygen combustion *free-radical exhaust* and the lack of a protective *telomere cap.*

mitochondrial biogenesis: In the capillary cell, this occurs because of the pendulum swing in combustion to nitric oxide, whose production becomes dependent on reductions in capillary-cell outer-membrane permeability caused by reductions in vascular inflammatory free radicals within the interstitial space.

mitochondrial combustion: A process that is oxygen dependent and, when healthy, pendulum swings back and forth from energy to nitric oxide production.

mitochondrial DNA: Naked (lacking *telomere caps*), it lies in the *mitochondrial matrix*. It supplies genetic coding for many of the proteins found in the *cytochrome system*.

mitochondrial exhaust: Is the exhaust from combustion of energy or nitric oxide.

mitochondrial fission: A process in which mitochondria decrease their volumes in a cell through *autophagocytosis*. This contraction of mitochondrial volumes occurs when there is too much combustion to make energy and not enough pendulum swing to make nitric oxide. This typically occurs in chronic inflammatory conditions in the interstitial space of end organs. As *superoxide* degrades mitochondrial DNA, mitochondrial fission occurs, where pieces of mitochondria are cut off and autodigested. (Compare with **mitochondrial fusion.**)

mitochondrial fusion: The opposite of *fission*. Pieces of mitochondria, or in some cases entire mitochondria, fuse together to create larger, highly functioning mitochondria. These new mitochondria can then replicate to further increase mitochondrial volumes when nitric oxide combustion is occurring. (Compare with **mitochondrial fission.**)

mitochondrial respiration: Another term for *mitochondrial combustion*.

mitochondrial transition pore: A large "suicide" pore originating in the *mitochondrial matrix* that signals imminent death of the mitochondria. This generally occurs if/when the *mitochondrial DNA* can no longer code effectively for protein synthesis because of too much free-radical damage.

mitophagy: Another term for the "suicide" created when mitochondria autodigest themselves.

mitosis: For purposes of this book, capillary cells may divide from growth factors. Mitochondria within capillary cells may increase their volumes through mitosis, which is facilitated by nitric oxide production.

monosaccharides: The most basic *carbohydrate* (single set of carbon rings), and contrasted with *disaccharides* (two sets of carbon rings), *trisaccharides* (three sets of carbon rings), and *polysaccharides* (multiple and branched sets of carbon rings). Polysaccharides, also known as *complex carbohydrates,* compose most plant fiber and are favorable to metabolism. Monosaccharides and disaccharides are simple and often refined sugars, are linked to vascular free radicals (AGEs) and are considered very vascular proinflammatory. (See also **disaccharides, polysaccharides,** and **trisaccharides**.)

monounsaturated fatty acids (MUFAs): These *monounsaturated oils* are very vascular anti-inflammatory and are found in avocados, olives, nuts, and dark chocolate. (See also **polyunsaturated fatty acids [PUFAs]**.)

morphology: Also known as *anatomic structure,* in this book, it refers to how capillary and end-organ cells have modified their outer membranes to accommodate specific end-organ function.

multiple sclerosis: Thought to be an *autoimmune disease* where immune proteins wrongly attack proteins found on axonal myelin sheaths of brain and spinal-cord cells. Progressive brain dysfunction at varying speeds of decline occurs.

myalgia: Also known as *skeletal-muscle pain,* this can be the result of infection in an end organ or skeletal muscle, statins, trauma, exercise, hypoxia, collagen vascular disease, peripheral vascular disease, malignancy, or kidney/liver failure.

myocardial infarction: Loss of heart muscle because of inadequate blood flow and oxygen support.

N-acetyl cysteine (NAC): An acetylated form of *cysteine* that is readily absorbable, has expanding medical benefits to preserving end-organ function, and can be utilized by end-organ and endothelial cells to make *glutathione,* an all-purpose *free-radical scavenger.*

N-acetylation: For purposes in this book, N-acetylation of *amino acids,* such as *cysteine,* can improve intestinal absorption.

naturopathic: A philosophy of medicine that utilizes natural substances, often plant based, to prevent and treat illnesses. Naturopathic treatments are expanding, as they appeal to a *holistic* sense of treatment benefit and are perceived to have fewer side effects.

nephron: The filtering unit of the *kidney,* which includes the *glomerulus* and a series of collecting tubules.

newer oral anticoagulants (NOACs): These are blood thinners, similar to Coumadin, that essentially block the vitamin K–driven coagulation cascade, thereby blocking the clotting cascade. This can treat and limits risks for *thrombosis.* In proinflammatory conditions where clots have caused or are causing a *hypoxic-ischemic event* (embolic TIA, CVA, deep vein thrombosis in the legs, or pulmonary embolus in the lung).

niacin: Vitamin B_3. Utilized as a cofactor in cellular operations; reduces blood LDL cholesterol and lipoprotein(a) in high doses.

nicotinamide: A congener of *niacin.* When ingested with vitamin D, it can lower skin cancer risk by up to 35 percent.

nicotinamide adenine dinucleotide (NAD/NADH): A congener of *niacin* (B_3) and an important hydrogen carrier in the *mitochondrial matrix.* From combinations of *pyruvate, beta-oxidation of fatty acids,* and *Krebs cycle metabolism,* hydrogen ions are released and couple with NAD (or FAD) to form NADH (or FADH). Both NADH and FADH transport *hydrogen* to the *cytochromes* of the *mitochondrial inner membrane,* where they uncouple to facilitate *electron transport* to make energy.

nicotinamide adenine dinucleotide phosphate (NADP/NADPH): A congener of *niacin* (B₃) and carries *hydrogen* utilized in the combustion of *mitochondrial nitric oxide.*

nicotinamide riboside (NR): A congener of *niacin,* nicotinamide riboside is a precursor in the production of NAD; therefore, increasing concentrations of NR facilitates NAD production and the subsequent hydrogen-carrying capacity within mitochondria to make energy. The theory is that the more hydrogen mitochondria can carry to the *cytochromes,* the more energy that can be produced.

nitrate: An ingested *nitroglycerin* that utilizes an alternative pathway to nitric oxide synthetase in mitochondria to make nitric oxide.

nitric oxide (NO): A gas molecule that causes smooth muscle of arteries to relax, dilating their *lumens* and increasing blood flow through them. Most nitric oxide in capillary and endothelial cells is synthesized from *arginine, citrulline,* and the enzyme *nitric oxide synthetase.* Mitochondrial nitric oxide production is part of the pendulum-swing feedback loop and increases when outer-membrane permeability decreases to inflammatory mediators. Nitric oxide is the rejuvenating gas, as it is linked to increased capillary-cell protein synthesis, and to repair and replacement of outer-membrane receptors, mitochondria, and nuclear telomeres. With age and chronic inflammation in the interstitial space of end organs, nitric oxide production decreases.

noradrenaline (catechomine): A stress hormone produced primarily in the adrenal glands.

nuclear DNA: DNA whose origin is from the *nucleus,* as opposed to *mitochondrial DNA.* Chromosomal nuclear DNA does have a *telomere cap* for protection.

nuclear imaging: Testing in which radioactive materials are injected or ingested, and then pictures of a specific organ are taken as the radioactive material accumulates in the organ studied, yielding an image that helps to determine pathology. Nuclear imaging can have an advantage to CT or MRI imaging in that it can approximate *function* of the end organ.

nucleus: The brain of the cell, it contains *chromosomal DNA* and a *nucleolus,* the latter of which is where DNA from the nucleus is copied in preparation for protein synthesis or cell division.

obesity: A *body mass index* (BMI) of 30–35. A BMI of 36 or higher is considered morbidly obese. One-third of adult Americans are obese, and up to one-fourth are morbidly obese.

obstructive plaque: The progressive development, usually in larger arterial vessels, of a *chronic cascading inflammatory plume* consisting of *cholesterol, calcium, platelets, cytokines,* and decomposed *white blood cells.* Over time a plaque can impinge and narrow the *vessel lumen* to cause an *occlusive thrombosis* in which blood flow is cut off upstream, jeopardizing the upstream end organ to a *hypoxic-ischemic event.* Obstructive plaques may also rupture, which cascades other serious conditions.

obstructive sleep apnea: An abnormal sleep pattern often directly linked to *obesity,* characterized by excessive snoring, airway obstruction, breathing irregularities with sleep, *hypoxia* when sleeping, brain fog, and excessive daytime drowsiness.

occlusion: Refers to blood flow cutoff in an artery or vein because of a *thrombosis* (clot) or an embolus (a piece of clot coming from elsewhere) in a vessel that is in spasm, is partially occluded by plaque, or has anatomical features conducive to occlusion.

occult: Hidden or stealth.

omega-3 fatty acids: Short- or long-chain fatty acids that have vascular anti-inflammatory properties.

omega-6 fatty acids: Long-chain fatty acids that can have vascular proinflammatory properties.

oncotic pressure: The pressure in blood vessels exerted by albumin that tends to "pull" water into the blood vessel from the interstitial space and endothelial and capillary cells. The effect is to limit risks for edema fluid in the interstitial space. (Compare with **osmotic pressure**.)

opioids: A class of pain medications, also known as *narcotics*, which can be dangerous to use because of abuse, addiction, tolerance to their effects, side effects, and increased risk for other vascular proinflammatory behaviors.

organelles: The internal "organs" of the cell. They have specific functions that feed back to each other. For the purposes of this book, examples of organelles include the *mitochondria, nucleus, ribosomes,* and the *rough and smooth endoplasmic reticulum.*

osmotic pressure: The pressure exerted on one side of a membrane to stop the "pull" or flow of a molecule to the other side. (Compare with **oncotic pressure**.)

osteoporosis: Occurs when the *bone matrix* thins or softens from loss of calcium. Osteoporosis causes bone pain, increases risk for bone fractures, and causes loss of height and change in posture.

outer membranes: A term used in this book to primarily refer to *capillary-cell outer membranes,* which include the *glycocalyx* (luminal side), *continuous outer membrane,* and *basement membrane* (abluminal side).

oxidation: A term used in reference to *mitochondrial respiration,* where oxygen is utilized to combust energy or nitric oxide. Oxidation generates *free radicals* that can endanger DNA and cellular infrastructure. *Oxidized small-particle LDL cholesterol* is highly inflammatory to endothelial- and capillary-cell outer membranes.

oxidative stress: The net accumulation of lingering *toxic free radicals* in the cell that endanger DNA, membranes, and organelles. Oxidative stress on capillary cells can occur from accumulation of vascular inflammatory free radicals (such as *LDL cholesterol, AGEs, tobacco toxins*) attached to their basement membranes to cause chronic inflammation, or can occur as free-radical exhaust (*superoxide*) from excessive energy combustion.

oxidized chain reactions: A process in which *free radicals* pass unstable electrons or protons to other molecules that would then make them free radicals. This is dangerous, as different types of free radicals create different kinds of damage to unsuspecting membranes, hence clustering inflammatory damage. The *antioxidants glutathione, vitamins C* and *E,* and *alpha-lipoic acid (ALA)* are examples of antioxidant team play, as they work together to prevent free-radical chain reactions.

oxygen: A ubiquitous and abundant atmospheric gas that is essential to human life and to mitochondrial combustion in all end organs, endothelial cells, and capillary cells.

oxygen tension: For the purposes of this book, this is the pressure that oxygen molecules exert as they diffuse in and out of *blood plasma, capillary cells,* the *interstitial space,* and the *end organ.*

Parkinson's syndrome: Also called *Parkinson's disease,* this is a movement disorder associated with resting tremors, shuffling gait, and cognitive decline (*dementia*); it is classified as a *neurodegenerative disorder.*

perfusion: An effect of *blood flow*. Blood flow to an end organ can increase or decrease, which increases or decreases exposure or perfusion to the end organ.

pericardium: The sac that contains the heart.

pericyte: A specialized *mural* or *helper cell* abutting the basement membrane of capillary cells in the interstitial space of end organs. Along with capillary and other *mesenchymal cells,* pericytes help maintain the integrity of the interstitial space of end organs.

periodontitis: Inflammation of the gum membrane often caused by bacteria and aggravated by sugary foods, leading to tooth decay, abscess, and loss of teeth. Bacteria from chronic periodontitis can enter the bloodstream and seed inflammation elsewhere, particularly on large-vessel endothelial-cell basement membranes supplying heart muscle and the brain.

peripheral vessel (vascular) disease: Inflammation of any blood vessel in the arterial tree beyond the aorta and its primary branches. A common feature of peripheral vascular disease is *chronic vascular inflammation* driven by *vascular inflammatory free radicals*. Endothelial-cell basement-membrane thickening and obstructive plaque result, causing upstream end-organ hypoxic-ischemic symptoms. An example would be *claudification,* calf/leg cramps and pain caused by lack of blood flow to leg skeletal muscle.

permeability: For the purposes of this book, this is defined as the capacity of capillary-cell outer membranes to increase or decrease movement of *inside-out, second-line inflammatory mediators* (also known as *white blood cells, cytokines, complement, immunoglobulins,* and *platelets*) into the interstitial space of end organs to affect an inflammatory response, vascular inflammatory free radial seeds, or subsequent complications.

244

peroxidation: A potential vascular proinflammatory effect triggered by *free radicals*, whereby a free radical attacks a *lipid* (usually unsaturated and more unstable) on a membrane surface to chain-react an even more unstable fat molecule. As membranes become more unstable (more exposed charges), they lend themselves to attract more proinflammatory mediators, hence exponentially increasing more inflammation on the membrane surface.

peroxisome proliferator activated receptors (PPARs): A family of proteins—alpha, beta, delta, and gamma—that, when activated, sequence enzyme reactions that can have net vascular anti-inflammatory benefits.

peroxisome proliferator receptor gamma coactivator (PGC-1-alpha): An *enzyme* that helps controls *mitochondrial biogenesis* (increase in intracellular mitochondria mass/quantity). With the pendulum swing of mitochondrial combustion to nitric oxide, PGC-1 levels increase, favoring *mitochondrial replication* and increased volumes.

phosphorus: The second-most abundant mineral in the body, its levels can fluctuate with vitamin D deficiency, malnutrition, parathyroid disorders, or kidney failure. Phosphorus is critical to mitochondrial combustion to make energy (ADP to ATP).

phytoplankton: Microscopic, photosynthesizing organisms that are the foundation of fresh- and saltwater food webs.

plasma: The component of blood minus red blood cells.

plasma membrane: The outer membrane of capillary cells that forms the barrier between the blood and the capillary cell. It is composed of the *glycocalyx* and *continuous outer membrane* on the *luminal side* of the endothelial and capillary cell.

platelets: Cells made in the bone marrow that facilitate clotting.

platelet adhesion: An inflammatory process that encourages platelets to adhere to membrane surfaces.

platelet aggregation: An inflammatory process, similar to platelet adhesion, that promotes the accumulation of platelets with the intent to form a clot (*thrombosis*).

pleotropism: Also known as *pleotropic benefits/effects*, the process in which blocking an intended effect chain-reacts to confer multiple other "added-on" effects. Pleotropic effects can be vascular pro- or anti-inflammatory. An example is that of *statins,* where lowering LDL cholesterol reduces inflammation of vascular membrane surfaces, thereby chain-reacting benefits leading to reducing hypoxic-ischemic events to oxygen-sensitive end organs (brain and heart) as well as causing reductions in end-organ cancers or serious infections.

podocytes: Specialized *epithelial cells* in the *kidney glomerulus* that, in combination with capillary cells, *ultrafiltrate* plasma in the initial steps of making *urine.*

polysaccharides: *Complex carbohydrates* that, when branched (such as in plant fiber), confer vascular anti-inflammatory benefits, which begin by improving the *intestinal microbiome.* (See also **disaccharides, monosaccharides,** and **trisaccharides.**)

polyunsaturated fatty acids (PUFAs): Fatty acids that contain more than one carbon double bond. PUFAs that are found in cheap vegetable oils are proinflammatory, as they easily convert to trans fats when heated. Fish oil PUFAs are vascular anti-inflammatory. (See also **monounsaturated fatty acids [MUFAs].**)

progesterone: A female hormone whose blood levels fluctuate during the menstrual cycle and permanently diminish in menopause.

propionyl coenzyme A (CoA): A final *beta-oxidation* end product of odd-chained *fatty acids*. Odd-chained fatty acids are found primarily in plant fats. It is thought that producing more propionyl CoA, as opposed to *acetyl CoA,* may reduce *insulin resistance,* as mitochondria may preferentially combust more *pyruvate.*

prostacyclins: In the family of *prostaglandins,* prostacyclins, when produced by *endothelial cells,* are considered vascular anti-inflammatory, as they cause smooth-muscle cells to relax (increasing blood flow to capillaries). Prostacyclins also block adhesion of *platelets* to membrane surfaces, limiting clot formation. Prostacyclins are now being used to treat *pulmonary hypertension,* a dangerous condition that eventually leads to respiratory failure. *Endothelin* creates a check-and-balance system with prostacyclin, as it produces opposite effects. With aging and chronic inflammation, biases increase capillary- and endothelial-cell endothelin production and decrease prostacyclin production.

prostaglandins: A diversified group of lipid-soluble fatty acids that are called *eicosanoids.* Prostaglandins have two subderivatives: *prostacyclins* and *thromboxanes.* Prostacyclins cause *arterial lumens* to dilate and limit *platelet aggregation,* whereas thromboxanes (including endothelin) do the opposite.

protein: Composed of organized *amino acids* of different lengths, protein is an essential constituent building block in all cells. For long-term survival, along with *carbohydrates* and *fat,* protein must be ingested.

protein kinase A (PKA): A family of *enzymes* that are activated by *cylic AMP* (cAMP) and important in regulation of cellular *metabolism.*

pseudocapillarization: An effect on capillary-cell outer membranes resulting from *chronic inflammation* in the interstitial space of end organs. It is characterized by a loss of membrane receptors, voltage gradients, and pore diversity, and biases increases in capillary- and endothelial-cell permeability to inflammatory mediators entering the interstitial space. Pseudocapillarization punctuates a *blocked capillary-cell dance,* marks capillary-cell disability, and implies *interstitial-space chronic inflammation* and *end-organ dysfunction.*

pterostilbene: An *antioxidant* similar to and probably more potent than *resveratrol.*

pulmonary hypertension: Dangerous condition characterized by increased pressures in the lung circulation, often from COPD, pulmonary fibrosis, pulmonary hypertension, or pulmonary embolus.

pyruvate: Also called *pyruvic acid,* this is the basic energy substrate from *glucose,* utilized by mitochondria to make *acetyl CoA.*

reactive oxygen species (ROS): Also called *free radicals,* which occur as the result of *mitochondrial combustion.*

red blood cells: Cells made in bone marrow that carry oxygen on their *hemoglobin.*

redox balance: The process in which one molecule is *oxidized* (hydrogen removed, electron exposed, molecule becomes more unstable) at the same time another molecule is *reduced* (hydrogen added, molecule becomes stable). *Antioxidants* are the masters of redox balance, as they counterbalance the pro effects of free radicals, thereby preventing *free-radical chain reactions.*

reduction: A process in which a molecule becomes more stable, generally by adding hydrogen to an exposed electron.

resveratrol: An *antioxidant* found in the skins of red grapes that has *pleotropic vascular anti-inflammatory properties.*

rhabdomyolysis: The breakdown of muscle filaments with the subsequent leaking of muscle enzymes in the blood to potentially cause muscle pain, weakness, and kidney failure.

ribosomal RNA: A specialized RNA that facilitates protein synthesis in ribosomes.

sarcopenia: Also called *skeletal-muscle atrophy* and/or *muscle wasting,* this occurs as a result of advanced age, chronic inflammation, and/or lack of exercise. There is a reduction in skeletal-muscle filament mass, with subsequent reduction in power and endurance of the affected muscle. The loss of skeletal-muscle mass leads to increased risk for diabetes and accelerates posture and gait abnormalities.

shear stress/inflammation: Increased pressure on *arterial lumen* walls both caused and affected by hypertension. The greatest levels of shear stress occur at arterial vessel bifurcations, where an artery divides into two smaller arteries.

sinusoid: A group of liver *hepatocytes* in combination with capillary cells form a *liver sinusoid* that receives a unique mixture of blood from the portal vein (intestinal nutrient) and artery (oxygenated blood).

sirtuins: A group of at least seven enzymes that affect mitochondrial function. *Sirtuin 1* and *3* increase nitric oxide levels by inhibiting energy combustion. Much of the sirtuin family is considered to have anti-inflammatory benefits.

sleep efficiency: The quality of sleep. Exemplary sleep efficiency implies seven continuous hours of uninterrupted deep sleep, which allows the brain optimal time to detoxify and aggregate the previous day's conscious activities.

sleep hygiene: Behaviors that increase or decrease *sleep efficiency.* Good sleep hygiene includes going to bed at the same time each night, sleeping in a quiet environment, and eliminating all nocturnal distractions affecting sleep. It also implies limiting catnaps during the day.

solubility: The capacity of a molecule to move through a membrane. Molecules are *fat-* or *water-soluble*, or both. Lipid- or fat-soluble molecules pass through membranes more easily than water-soluble molecules.

somatic cells: In this book, somatic cells are defined as *end-organ epithelial cells*.

space of Disse: The *interstitial space* in the *liver sinusoid* between portal capillary cells and *hepatocytes*.

statins: A group of medications with origins to red rice yeast that lower LDL cholesterol and reduce vascular inflammation, thereby reducing vascular inflammatory free-radical burden on endothelial-cell basement membranes and in the interstitial space. Statins have *pleotropic effects* to chronic inflammation, meaning they reduce hypoxic-ischemic events, cancer, autoimmune-complex disease, and serious infections (sepsis). (See also **HMG-CoA reductase inhibitors**.)

stellate cells: Specialized *pericytes* found in the *space of Disse* in *liver sinusoids*.

succinyl coenzyme A (CoA): An end product in *beta-oxidation* of *fatty acids*.

superfoods: Whole, fresh foods, often from plants, that have abundant antioxidants, minerals, and complex carbohydrates and are considered very vascular anti-inflammatory.

superoxides: *Free radicals*, or ROS, generated from *mitochondrial energy combustion*. If they linger and are not neutralized, they cause damage to membrane surfaces and DNA.

tau: An amyloid-like substance that is secreted in the brain and is associated with *chronic vascular inflammation*, advanced forms of *dementia*, and *cerebral atrophy*.

telomere cap: The protective cap on *nuclear chromosomes* that prevents damage from *free radicals*. With age and chronic inflammation, nuclear telomeres shrink, thereby leading to more DNA cross-linkage from free radicals. Telomere caps regrow by the enzyme *telomerase*, which becomes active with a pendulum swing in mitochondrial combustion from energy to nitric oxide production. *Mitochondrial DNA* lacks a telomere cap.

testosterone: Male hormone produced in the testes in men. Small amounts are also produced in the female ovary.

thrombin: A proinflammatory mediator that increases clotting cascades.

thrombosis: When clotting cascades and *platelets* produce a *clot*. Thrombosis can be dangerous when it occludes arteries and cuts off blood supply to end organs upstream, thereby causing a *hypoxic-ischemic event* to the end organ.

thromboxanes: Potentially proinflammatory molecules that, when released by *platelets* or capillary cells promote, *coagulation* and constriction of blood vessels.

trans fat: An unstable vascular proinflammatory fat originating from polyunsaturated vegetable oils upon exposure to heat.

transient ischemic attack (TIA): Also known as a *ministroke*, this is the result of a *hypoxic-ischemic event* to the brain, where there is a transient loss of function (usually less than one hour) to specific parts of the brain because of blood flow cutoff, followed by recovery. TIAs are very dangerous, as one attack generally leads to more. If they accumulate in number, they can cause cognitive deficits similar to larger strokes. They are a stealth cause of *dementia*.

triglycerides: Complex *fat molecules* that, when elevated in the blood, are vascular proinflammatory. They can be increased from obesity, metabolic syndrome, diabetes, low thyroid conditions, fatty liver, or genetic predisposition. Exercise, plant fiber, weight loss, correction of thyroid conditions, treatment of diabetes, fish oil (EPA), and fibrates all lower blood triglycerides.

trisaccharides: Another type of *simple carbohydrate* that is vascular proinflammatory. (See also **disaccharides**, **monosaccharides**, and **polysaccharides**.)

tumor necrosis factor (TNF): Proinflammatory mediator.

ultrafiltrate: The end product after blood plasma has been filtered through the *glomerulus*.

ultrasound: Also known as *sonography*, this is noninvasive imaging that does not employ radiation or contrast dye. An excellent technique to screen for diseases, it can be used serially to assess changes in condition without radiation harm to the patient.

ureter: The tube that takes urine from the kidney pelvis to the bladder.

urethra: The tube that drains urine from the bladder.

vascular tone: The degree of responsiveness of a blood vessel's smooth muscle to relax or constrict in order to increase or decrease flow through the *arterial lumen*. Large-vessel plaque buildup or basement-membrane thickening blocks smooth-muscle responsiveness and decreases vascular tone.

vasoactive endothelial growth factor (VEGF): A *proinflammatory mediator* that is produced in response to hypoxic-ischemic events, infections, trauma, cancer, or other acute inflammatory conditions in the interstitial space of end organs.

ventilation: The process of breathing (inspiration and exhaling).

very low-density lipoprotein (VLDL cholesterol): Another inflammatory cholesterol that is part of the measurement of *non-HDL cholesterol*.

vesicles: Serve as *endothelial-* and *capillary-cell transporters*. In this book, they refer to active-transport processes, involving capillary-cell outer membranes, that mobilize proteins and inflammatory mediators to and from the blood to the interstitial space of end organs. The vesicle shuttle works best when there is adequate on-demand energy from adjacent mitochondria.

vitamins B, C, D, E, and K: Families of *essential vitamins* that are necessary for optimal cellular function.

VO₂ max: A measure of the volume of oxygen used with maximum exercise, it is the gold standard for measuring the capacity to exercise—that is, the higher the VO_2 max, the greater the exercise effort. Its measurement is generally confined to a physiology laboratory. An estimation of VO_2 max is the MET, which is utilized in most common exercise protocols as an estimate of exercise performance.

voltage gradient: The *electric current* that a membrane possesses. Higher-voltage gradients make penetration of molecules through the membrane more difficult. Voltage gradients are often increased from pumps involving sodium and potassium and decreased in the presence of calcium ions. The capillary-cell outer membrane of the blood-brain barrier has a higher-voltage gradient than capillary cells elsewhere. The higher gradient is one way that capillary cells provide additional barrier support to brain cells.

white blood cells: A family of inflammatory cells that are made in the bone marrow or lymph tissue and often stored in the spleen, have many different and specialized properties, and can be either pro- or anti-inflammatory, often influenced by *chronic interstitial-space inflammation* from *vascular inflammatory free-radical seeds*.

Appendix

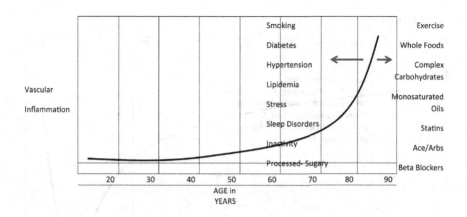

Graph 1

Endothelial- or Capillary-Cell Inflammation/Dysfunction, Aging Acceleration, and Reversal

This graph depicts common proinflammatory vascular-mediator risks (also known as vascular inflammatory free radicals) and how they shift the aging curve to the left to accelerate aging by increasing chronic inflammation within the interstitial spaces of end organs. To the right of the curve are behaviors, dietary interventions, and selected treatments that reduce chronic interstitial-space inflammation and shift the aging curve to the right to lengthen life and reduce pain and fatigue.

(Courtesy of R. Buckingham, *Hazing Aging*, Bloomington, IN: iUniverse, 2015)

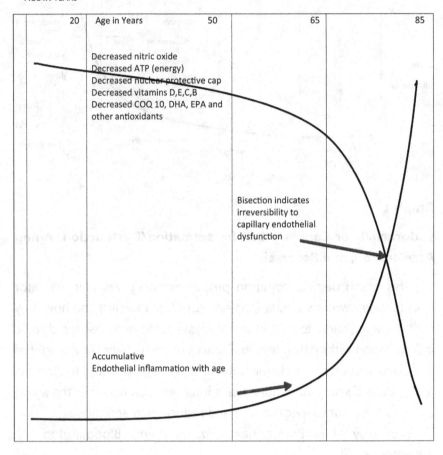

The labels within the graph read:

| 20 | Age in Years | 50 | 65 | 85 |

Decreased nitric oxide
Decreased ATP (energy)
Decreased nuclear protective cap
Decreased vitamins D,E,C,B
Decreased COQ 10, DHA, EPA and
other antioxidants

Bisection indicates
irreversibility to
capillary endothelial
dysfunction

Accumulative
Endothelial inflammation with age

Graph 2

Age-Accumulative Endothelial- or Capillary-Cell Inflammation and Changes in Endothelial-Cell Markers of Function

These lines in the graph, as they converge and bisect, indicate more-rapid and then terminal end-organ declines from a persistently blocked back-and-forth swinging of a capillary-cell outer-membrane permeability pivot and mitochondrial combustion pendulum swing. The top line represents age-related declines in mitochondrial volumes as measured by nitric oxide and energy combustion linked to increased ROS, exhausted antioxidants, and depleted vitamin cofactors. The bottom line represents increasing and chronic interstitial-space

258

inflammation in end organs. As chronic interstitial-space inflammation increases, capillary- and endothelial-cell outer-membrane permeability fluxing is blocked, which then feeds back to prevent the mitochondrial combustion swing to the rejuvenating nitric oxide. At a critical point (where the two lines in the graph bisect), the combination of chronic interstitial-space inflammation and the blocked capillary-cell dance causes capillary cells to become irreversibly dysfunctional. This completes the stage of anti-organ interstitial space preeminence, where numerous venues have been created to disrupt the interstitial space and isolate and decay the end organ. Residuals from venues include interstitial-space scarring, incremental growth of cancer(s), the emergence of superinfections and sepsis, umerous rogue autoimmune complexes, and thrombotic-hypoxic-ischemic events. As end organs decline, fatigue and pain increase. Beyond the bisected lines, to the far right of the graph, are the inevitable capillary cell and end organ)s) failures culminating in death.

(Courtesy of R. Buckingham, *Hazing Aging*, Bloomington, IN: iUniverse, 2015)

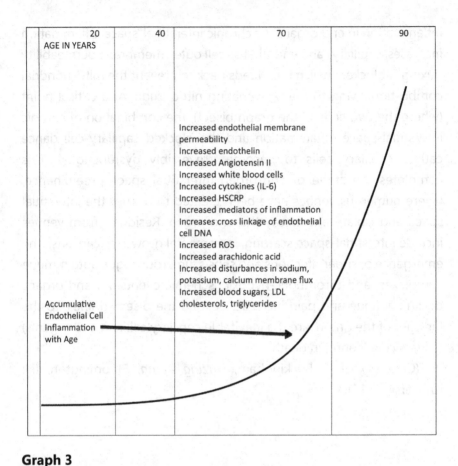

Graph 3

Endothelial- or Capillary-Cell Inflammation and Markers of Chronic Inflammation, with Age

This graph depicts the relationship of chronic interstitial-space inflammation, vascular inflammatory seeding by free radicals, pluming of immune arsenal (white blood cells, cytokines, and other inflammatory mediators) and its progression to eventually block the capillary cell outer membrane mitochondrial dance. Without the capillary dance that fuels rejuvenation, capillary cells don't replace outer-membrane receptors or replenish mitochondrial volumes, nuclear telomeres or its infrastructure which ultimately dooms them to fail. As they fail, they take their interstitial space partner mesenchymal and end organ cells with them. This is because they won't and can't seed or pace rejuvenation to either mesenchymal or end organ cells. As this collapsing relationship occurs between capillary and end organ cells various inflammatory markers, as depicted in the graph, increase in the bloodstream. These markers predict declines and accelerated aging of the end organ, chronic illnesses within the interstitial spaces of end organs, and increases in fatigue and pain.

(Courtesy of R. Buckingham, *Hazing Aging*, Bloomington, IN: iUniverse, 2015)

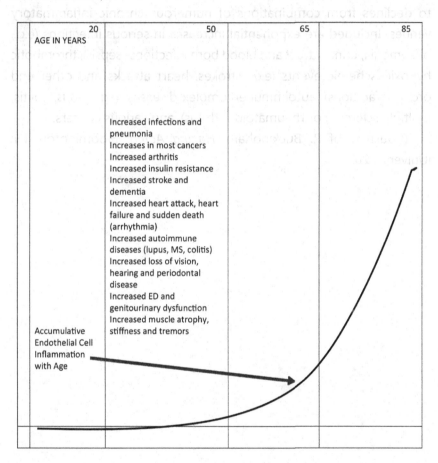

Graph 4

Chronic End-Organ Interstitial-Space Inflammation, Aging, and Increased Expression of Diseases

Because of chronic inflammation in the interstitial space of end organs (induced and perpetuated by vascular inflammatory free-radical seeds), capillary-cell outer membranes and mitochondria do not dance. The fall-out of this block is the inability for endothelial and capillary cells to rejuvenate. This causes reduced endothelial and capillary cell mitochondrial volumes, pseudocapillarization of outer membranes, and shortened nuclear telomeres. As capillary cells decline in function, the interstitial spaces of end organs become at risk for more immune arsenal mistakes. Eventually this culminates in end organ vulnerability to declines from combinations of numerous chronic inflammatory venues. Included are exponential increases in serious infections (e.g., pneumonia, urinary tract and blood born infections- sepsis), thrombotic hypoxic-ischemic events (e.g., strokes. heart attacks and other end organ infarctions), autoimmune-complex diseases (e.g., lupus, colitis, multiple sclerosis, or rheumatoid arthritis), and various cancers.

(Courtesy of R. Buckingham, *Hazing Aging*, Bloomington, IN: iUniverse, 2015)

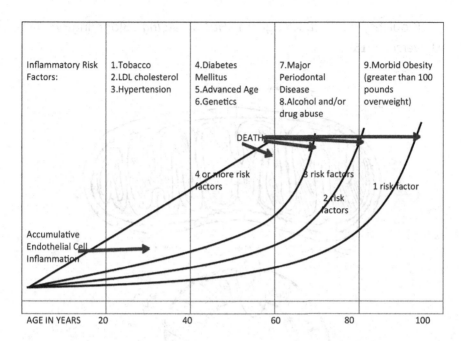

| Inflammatory Risk Factors: | 1.Tobacco 2.LDL cholesterol 3.Hypertension | 4.Diabetes Mellitus 5.Advanced Age 6.Genetics | 7.Major Periodontal Disease 8.Alcohol and/or drug abuse | 9.Morbid Obesity (greater than 100 pounds overweight) |

DEATH

4 or more risk factors

3 risk factors

2 risk factors

1 risk factor

Accumulative Endothelial Cell Inflammation

AGE IN YEARS 20 40 60 80 100

Graph 5

Effect of Endothelial- or Capillary-Cell Inflammation and Stacking of Free-Radical Inflammatory Risk Factors on Mortality, with Age

This graph correlates the stacking of untreated vascular inflammatory free radicals, chronic interstitial-space inflammation, and the subsequent acceleration of aging and death that occurs from inflammatory free-radical stacking over time. As an example, having just one inflammatory free radical risk factor of the nine depicted in the graph does little to shift the mortality curve to shorten life expectancy. However, vascular inflammatory free radicals can be very addictive and have a propensity to attract behaviors leading to more free radicals. When combinations occur, such as tobacco smoke toxins, elevated blood sugars (adult diabetes) and LDL cholesterol, the impact on life expectancy is substantial. The mortality curve shifts dramatically to shortened life spans with more pain and fatigue. Having four or more untreated vascular inflammatory risk factors can shorten life expectancy by twenty-five or more years! Fatigue and pain often precede death by 10 years meaning that 35 years or more of life have been either cut short or tormented.

(Courtesy of R. Buckingham, *Hazing Aging*, Bloomington, IN: iUniverse, 2015)

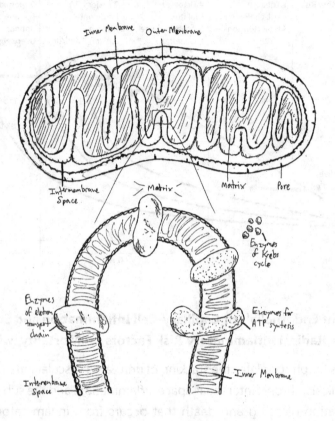

Figure 1

Anatomy of Capillary Mitochondria

Capillary mitochondria are composed of a porous outer membrane, intermembrane space (where hydrogen ions are stored), inner membrane (where the cytochrome clumps of proteins pass electrons), and a core matrix (where calcium ions are stored, naked mitochondrial DNA is found, and mitochondrial combustion infrastructure is housed).

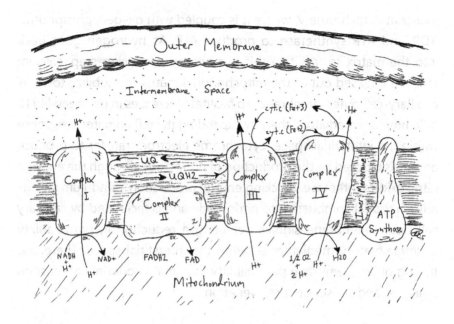

Figure 2

The Movement of Hydrogen Ions (H+) from the Matrix to the Intermembrane Space of Mitochondria

This figure highlights the five cytochrome complexes on the mitochondrial inner membrane, depicting how the cytochromes receive hydrogen ions from NADH and FADH. As they facilitate electron transfer, they are spit into the intermembrane space. The gap of hydrogen between the mitochondrial matrix and intermembrane space helps to creates the potent inner-membrane voltage gradient. Electron transfer through the cytochromes is facilitated by metal cations such as the heme (iron [Fe]) ring. As electrons are passed down a string of metal cations within the cytochromes, hydrogen is released into the intermembrane space where it fortifies the powerful inner-membrane voltage gradient. The potent voltage gradient produces tight control of what goes in and comes out of the mitochondrial matrix. As being the mother of all membrane voltage gradients, it facilitates feedback loop control to other membranes and organelles. The accumulated hydrogen within the intermembrane space is eventually released back into the matrix at cytochrome V, where it is coupled with oxygen, phosphorus, ADP, and ATP synthetase to produce ATP. As hydrogen goes back into the matrix to facilitate this last energy producing step, calcium ions are released out of the mitochondrial matrix to mobilize towards capillary-cell outer membranes to facilitate increases in permeability to inflammatory mediators, thereby expanding the inflammatory response within the interstitial space. Cytochrome electron transfer to produce energy is blocked by the production of nitric oxide through the enzyme nitric oxide synthetase. Blocking energy production, pendulum swings mitochondrial combustion to nitric oxide and is facilitated by capillary cell outer membrane signals depicting a reduction in permeability to inflammatory mediators entering the interstitial space. Therefore, fluxing outer membrane permeability keys mitochondrial combustion swinging and subsequent rejuvenation.

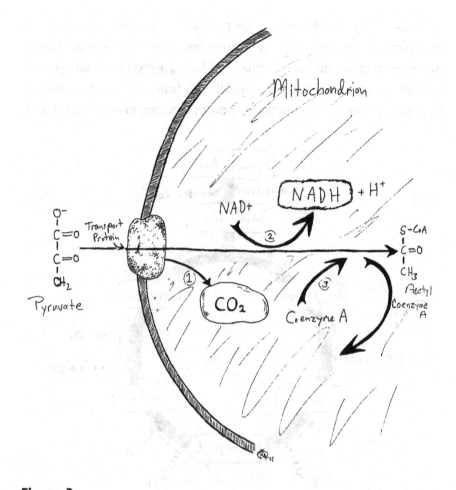

Figure 3

Production of Acetyl Coenzyme A from Pyruvate in the Mitochondrial Matrix

Pyruvate is produced from glucose in the endothelial and capillary cell's cytoplasm through anaerobic glycolysis and enters the mitochondrial matrix by a transport protein through the inner membrane. Once in the matrix, in just a single enzyme step, coenzyme A and sulfur (S) are added to the molecule to make acetyl CoA. During the process of making acetyl CoA, hydrogen (H) is released to NAD to form NADH. NADH becomes a hydrogen transporter, depositing the hydrogen into the cytochrome system of electron transfer. In the meantime, acetyl CoA can be utilized in the Krebs cycle for energy combustion or be transported to ribosomes or rough endoplasmic reticulum during mitochondrial nitric oxide combustion to make new proteins during rejuvenation. Making acetyl CoA from pyruvate (as compared to fatty-acid beta-oxidation) is faster, and because there is just one enzymatic step, over time produces less toxic free-radical exhaust.

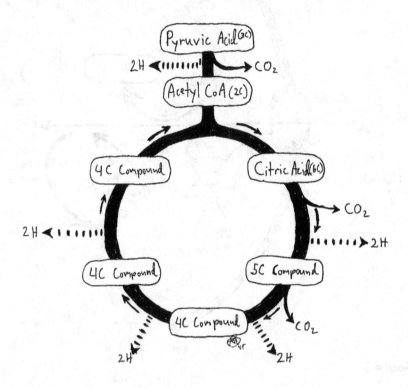

Figure 4

Pyruvic Acid (Pyruvate) Entering the Krebs Cycle

After pyruvate (pyruvic acid) becomes acetyl CoA, it can enter the Krebs cycle (also known as the *citric* acid cycle). In the Krebs cycle, acetyl CoA is eventually catabolized (broken down to basic molecules) to cause release of hydrogen, carbon dioxide, water (and occasionally other exhausts) and ATP energy (not shown). The abundant hydrogen ion (H) booty from catabolized acetyl CoA is picked up by NAD and FAD transporters and deposited at the cytochromes, where it facilitates electron transport. All these steps augment mitochondrial energy combustion, which in capillary cells supports increased permeability and subsequent active transport of inflammatory mediators into the interstitial space to hopefully resolve inflammatory breach.

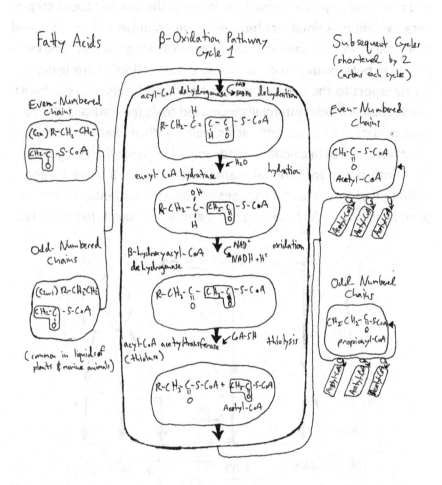

Figure 5

Acetyl Coenzyme A Production from Fatty-Acid Beta-Oxidation

In capillary mitochondria, acetyl CoA, which is the hub of mitochondrial combustion, can be produced from pyruvate, fatty acids, or ketone bodies, the latter of which is produced in the liver from fatty acids as a result of starvation or from very low calorie diets. Beta-oxidation of fatty acids in capillary and endothelial cells differs from pyruvate metabolism in that several enzymes and metabolic steps are required to process fatty-acid chains. Odd-number carbon chains, found in vegetable fats, produce one acetyl CoA molecule and one propionyl coenzyme A molecule in the last metabolic step of beta oxidation. Animal fats have only even numbers of carbons and therefore produce two acetyl CoA molecules in the last step. The extra step(s) in beta-oxidation of fatty acid chains yield(s) more hydrogen for transport to the cytochromes but also produce(s) more exhaust, which could include potentially increased toxic free radicals. Because beta oxidation of plant fatty acids yields a diversified end product, plant fatty acid beta oxidation tends to trickle rather than surge acetyl Co A into the mitochondrial matrix. This enables a more balanced utilization of pyruvate which causes less insulin resistance. That means plant fats lessen risks towards adult diabetes compared to animal fats.

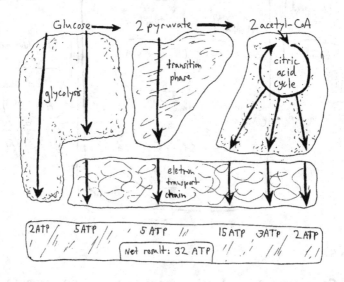

Figure 6

Glucose to Pyruvate to Acetyl Coenzyme A Metabolism and Energy Yields

Glucose can enter capillary cells and be converted to pyruvate by anaerobic glycolysis in the cell's cytoplasm. Glycolysis can yield a small amount of ATP, but also produces two pyruvate molecules from one glucose molecule. Pyruvate can be transported into the mitochondrial matrix to be quickly reduced to two acetyl CoA molecules. Acetyl CoA can enter the Krebs cycle or be shuttled to ribosomes for protein synthesis. When acetyl CoA is catabolized in the Krebs cycle, it generates a small amount of ATP, but releases large quantities of hydrogen ion, which becomes the primary facilitator of hydrogen to the cytochrome electron transport chain as well as creating the inner membrane voltage gradient. In the last cytochrome (cytochrome V), hydrogen is removed from the intermembrane space and reintroduced back into the mitochondrial matrix, where in the presence of ATP synthetase, oxygen, ADP, and phosphorus, converts ADP to ATP. One glucose molecule, when utilized to combust energy in the mitochondrial matrix, eventually yields thirty-two ATP molecules, with most of the yield coming from electron transfer and cytochrome V.

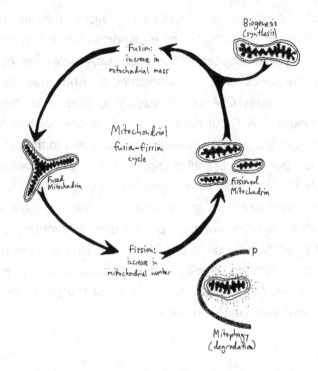

Figure 7

Fluctuations in Capillary-Cell Mitochondrial Volumes from Pro- or Anti-inflammatory Influences

This figure depicts the real time life cycles of capillary-cell mitochondria and how their volumes within a capillary cell can flux based on the presence of chronic end-organ interstitial-space inflammation. Blocking the capillary-cell dance (outer-membrane permeability pivot and mitochondrial combustion pendulum swing) persistently increases mitochondrial energy combustion and subsequent superoxide free-radical exhaust. The superoxide perpetuation exhausts antioxidants to eventually bind to mitochondrial membrane surfaces and naked DNA to result in increased mitochondrial incompetence. The silencing of mitochondrial function from DNA incompetence increases mitochondrial fission (amputation) and suicide (mitophagy). This reduces capillary cell mitochondrial volumes and keys capillary cell pseudocapillarization of outer membranes, leading to the dispensation of the anti-organ interstitial space venues. On the other hand, by reducing vascular inflammatory free radical seeding within the interstitial space, the opposite occurs. The capillary-cell dance resumes, mitochondrial combustion swing to nitric oxide and capillary-cell rejuvenation returns in earnest. Without energy combustion, superoxide free radicals decrease in the mitochondrial matrix enabling mitochondria to fuse and replicate (biogenesis). This has the effect of increasing their volumes in capillary cells, which can then d rive reversal of outer membrane pseudocapillarization, as there is more energy available to support pore diversity, voltage gradients and outer membrane receptors. Whether capillary mitochondria fission, fuse or replicate is dependent on inflammatory momentum within the interstitial space.

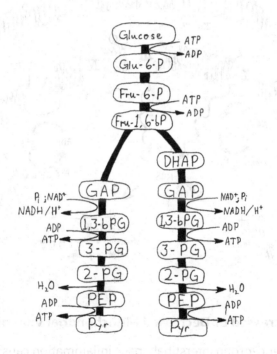

Figure 8

Glycolysis

Glycolysis in capillary cells occurs in their cytoplasm. It takes glucose and, in a methodical ten-step process, and converts it to two pyruvate molecules without the use of oxygen (also known as anaerobic metabolism or fermentation). The production of pyruvate by glycolysis (as well as its reverse, gluconeogenesis) becomes an important feedback loop in the management of energy-substrate homeostasis within capillary-cell mitochondria. When pyruvate utilization by mitochondria decreases (as when there is abundant fatty acid substrate), pyruvate can be transported back to the cytoplasm and be converted to glucose (gluconeogenesis). In this fashion, the refinement of mitochondrial energy substrate homeostasis is facilitated by its feedback-loop relationships with glycolysis and gluconeogenesis.

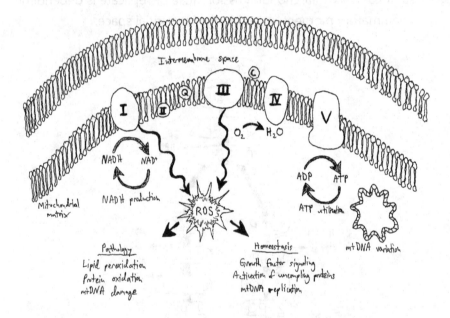

Figure 9

ROS and Increased or Decreased Mitochondrial Volumes

Chronic end-organ interstitial-space inflammation causes capillary-cell mitochondria to combust more energy, thereby creating more superoxide (ROS) free-radical exhaust. As depicted previously the superoxide exhaust damages mitochondrial DNA to cause reduction in their volumes in the capillary cell. Superoxide damage can spread to involve capillary-cell infrastructure and nuclear DNA. This ROS effect is depicted in the figure as combinations of membrane lipid (fatty acid) and protein peroxidation occurs from a combination of a direct disruptive effect ROS has when attached to membrane surfaces as well as an indirect effect it has from silencing membrane protein function on the basis of defective protein synthesis from malfunctioning cross-linked nuclear DNA. With a return of the capillary-cell dance, nitric oxide combustion rejuvenates could help reverse this dark slide as superoxide combustion exhaust dries up. This swing of mitochondrial combustion allows for repletion of over utilized antioxidants such as glutathione and MnSOD. Rejuvenating these antioxidants as well as others, limits free radical collateral damage by reducing free radical chain reactions.

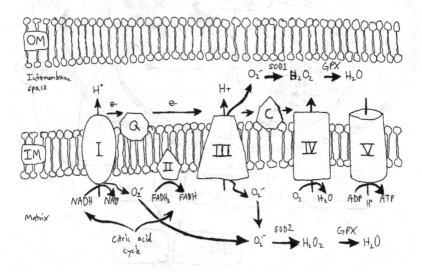

Figure 10

The Importance of Antioxidants—SOD

In this figure, mitochondrial energy combustion, through the passage of electrons in cytochromes, causes production of superoxide free-radical exhaust. Lingering superoxide (O2-) can produce damage to DNA and membrane surfaces and must be reduced by glutathione and SOD (also known as MnSOD, manganese superoxide dismutase). At the bottom of the figure, SOD2 (superoxide dismutase two) reduces superoxide to hydrogen peroxide, which is then further reduced by GPX (glutathione peroxidase) to water. When mitochondrial nitric oxide combustion is stimulated, the cytochrome passage of electrons is blocked, and superoxide ROS production decreases. This allows for the replenishment of SOD and glutathione antioxidants.

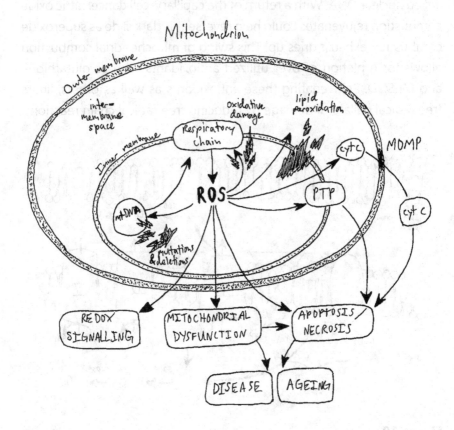

Figure 11

The Damaging Effects of ROS Exhaust Coming from Excessive Mitochondrial Energy Combustion

This figure demonstrates how mitochondrial ROS exhaust can cluster cell damage. As capillary-cell mitochondria produce energy and release calcium ions to support active transport of immune arsenal into the interstitial space, more superoxide ROS exhaust is produced. Superoxide produces oxidative stress on membranes by causing lipid peroxidation. It can damage DNA through cross-linkage, thereby producing chromosomal mutations and deletions, which cause defective coding of proteins. ROS can even have an effect on redox signaling, which can induce a series of proinflammatory chain reactions within the capillary cell. Since age and chronic inflammation biases mitochondrial combustion toward more energy and less nitric oxide, superoxide toxic exhaust tends to increase. The blocked capillary-cell pivot and pendulum-swing dance, caused from chronic vascular inflammatory seeding of the interstitial space, becomes the linchpin to excessive superoxide ROS exhaust.

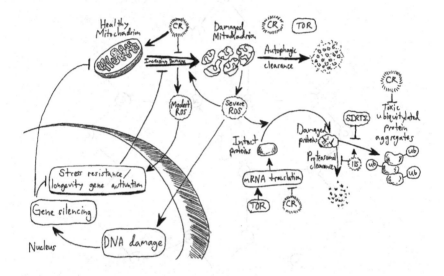

Figure 12

Redox Signaling of Mitochondrial ROS

Superoxide ROS accumulates based on mitochondrial energy combustion and is caused by a combination of overproduction and overutilization of antioxidants (MnSOD, glutathione). Superoxide exhaust can actually be helpful in mitigating an acute inflammatory breach, as it amplifies the inflammatory response to help cause resolution of the breach. It is in chronic inflammation of the interstitial space where superoxide free radicals turn from friend to foe. In this setting, superoxide causes membrane lipid peroxidation and cross-links mitochondrial and nuclear DNA (see figure), which can subsequently silence the expression of genes, favoring the coding of incompetent essential proteins, and inducing their silent functioning. Eventually, as more proteins become silent (and mitochondrial volumes shrink) the capillary cell functions as shell. In this phase of rapid decline, end-organ function deteriorates quickly as the anti-organ implements its different cascades of antagonistic venues.

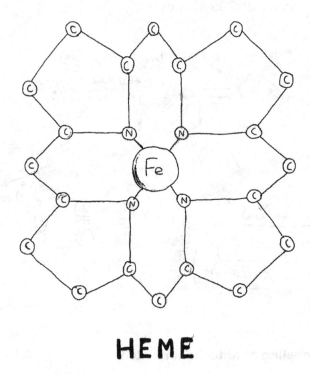

HEME

Figure 13

Heme Molecule

Heme is essentially a ring of carbons encircling iron. In the endothelial and capillary cell, heme is critical to electron transfer through the cytochromes. The production of heme is complex, involves feedback loops from the capillary cell cytoplasm and adjacent smooth endoplasmic reticulum, and is controlled by rate limiting enzymes within the mitochondrial matrix. Heme homeostasis is counterbalanced by heme *catabolism* (breakdown), which occurs primarily in the adjacent smooth endoplasmic reticulum. Both heme production and catabolism are dependent on feedback loops related to what kind of capillary cell mitochondrial combustion is occurring. Heme homeostasis is disturbed with a blocked capillary cell dance.

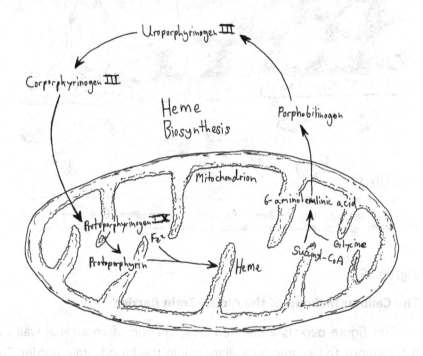

Figure 14

Mitochondrial Heme Production

Heme production involves enzymes and intermediates that cycle into and out of the mitochondria. Heme synthesis begins with succinyl coenzyme A and glycine in the mitochondrial matrix. After three production steps in the mitochondrial matrix, heme metabolism moves into the cytoplasm to involve several more steps before reentering the matrix to complete production. As previously mentioned Heme homeostasis is regulated by feedback loops involving mitochondrial energy and nitric oxide combustion, the facilitation of production enzymes within the cytoplasm and subsequent catabolism of heme back to its individual components in the smooth endoplasmic reticulum.

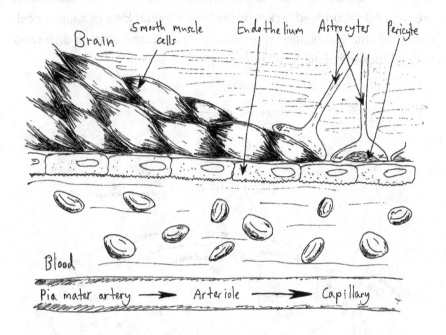

Figure 15

The Cellular Makeup of the Blood-Brain Barrier

This figure depicts a blended cross section of an arterial wall as it transitions to become a capillary cell in the blood-brain barrier. To the left of the figure are arteriole endothelial cells that are encircled by smooth muscle. The smooth muscle responds to nitric oxide and other substances to either relax or slide (contract) their actin-myosin filaments, to cause relaxation or constriction of the vessel lumen, thereby increasing or decreasing blood flow through the vessel and to the capillary cells of the blood-brain barrier. Although total blood flow to the brain remains constant, adjustments in blood flow to different regions of the brain to accommodate different cerebral functions is facile and dependent on how well arterioles respond to dilating and constricting influences. Arterioles transition in the figure to capillary cells, which along with astrocytes and pericytes, form the blood-brain barrier. Together they produce an ultra -strict barrier that prevents most blood plasma constituents from having access to brain nerve cells. In contrast to capillary cells elsewhere, capillary cells of the blood-brain barrier are tightly compacted, with very tight gap junctions. This helps to seal off any chance that blood constituents might have to leak into the cerebrospinal fluid (CSF). With chronic inflammation and the perpetuation of vascular free-radical seeding in end organ interstitial spaces, even the blood-brain barrier is breached, causing increased exposures to the brain of inflammatory constituents. The most common type of outcome to chronic interstitial space inflammation in the brain is progressive dementia, and is attributable to chronic inflammatory venues that include thrombosis and interstitial space amyloid and tau scarring with the subsequent development of cerebral trophy.

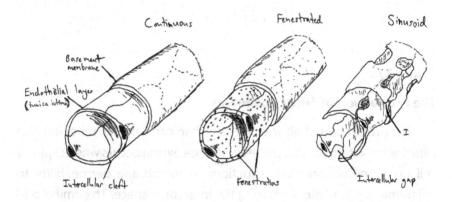

Figure 16

Different Capillary-Cell Outer-Membrane Morphologies

This figure demonstrates the different appearances of capillary-cell basement membranes and continuous outer membranes based on where capillary cells reside. To the far left of the figure is the capillary-cell outer membrane in the blood-brain barrier. The basement membrane is tightly compacted, with no gaps. In the far right, the capillary-cell basement membrane in the liver sinusoid is the opposite. It is loosely fitted, with large gaps and multiple pores, or fenestrae. Examples of the middle capillary cell, where there are many pores but no gaps in the basement membranes, may be found in the kidney glomerulus or intestine.

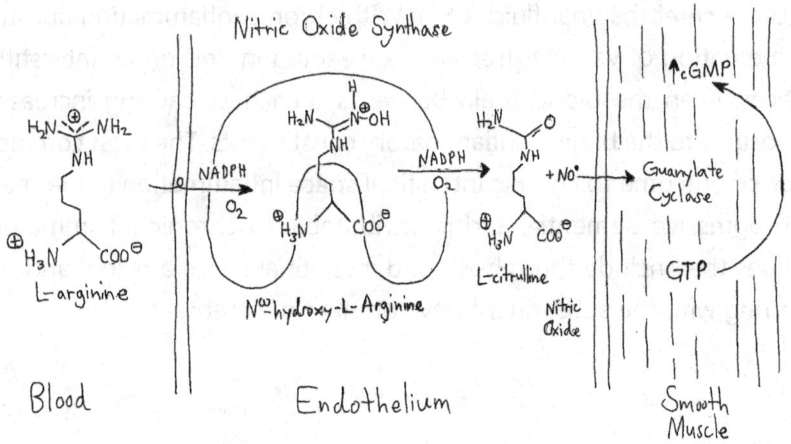

Nitric Oxide Synthase

L-arginine

N$^\omega$-hydroxy-L-Arginine

L-citrulline

Nitric Oxide

Guanylate Cyclase

$\uparrow$cGMP

GTP

Blood

Endothelium

Smooth Muscle

Figure 17

The Production of Nitric Oxide Gas

The production of nitric oxide begins in capillary cell mitochondria with the activation of nitric oxide synthetase, which occurs when capillary cell outer membrane flux reductions in membrane permeability to inflammatory mediators entering the interstitial space. The amino acid L-arginine is then signaled to enters the endothelial and capillary cell mitochondria and, with combinations of oxygen, NADPH, and activated nitric oxide synthetase, is converted to citrulline and nitric oxide gas. Citrulline can be recycled to regenerate L-arginine, while nitric oxide gas diffuses through membrane surfaces to switch on capillary cell rejuvenation while also entering the circulation to cause relaxation of arteriole smooth muscle by increasing the conversion of GTP to GMP. Activation of nitric oxide synthetase is a powerful blocker to mitochondrial ATP combustion and all the *feedback* sub loops that proceed from it.

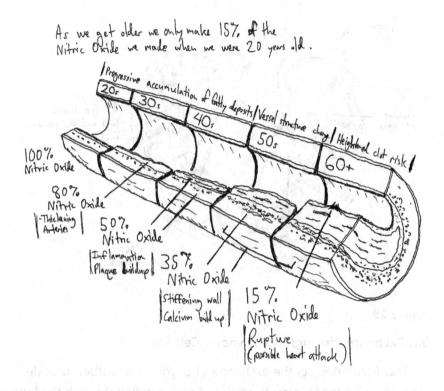

As we get older we only make 15% of the Nitric Oxide we made when we were 20 years old.

Progressive accumulation of fatty deposits / Vessel structure change / Heightened clot risk

20s 30s 40s 50s 60+

100% Nitric Oxide

80% Nitric Oxide
|-Thickening Arteries|

50% Nitric Oxide
|Inflammation Plaque buildup|

35% Nitric Oxide
|Stiffening wall Calcium build up|

15% Nitric Oxide
|Rupture (possible heart attack)|

Figure 18

The Cause and Effect of Large-Vessel Obstructive Plaque on Nitric Oxide Production

Nitric oxide homeostasis by endothelial and capillary cell mitochondria s is directly dependent on how much chronic inflammation is occurring within their interstitial spaces and the volume of large-vessel obstructive plaque that has occurred in downstream arterial vessels. The chronic narrowing of large vessel lumens downstream reduces blood flow to upstream capillaries creating more oxidative stress on them thereby producing biases towards more energy and less nitic oxide production. As plaque grows, nitric oxide production in upstream capillaries sharply diminishes.

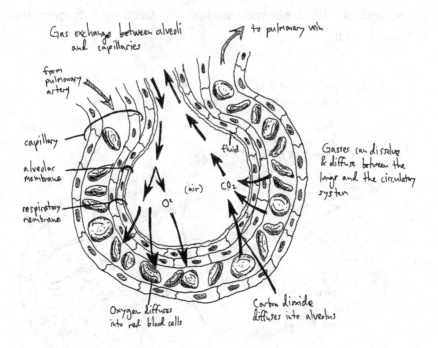

Gas exchange between alveoli and capillaries

to pulmonary vein

from pulmonary artery

capillary

alveolar membrane

respiratory membrane

fluid

(air)   O₂   CO₂

Gasses can dissolve & diffuse between the lungs and the circulatory system

Oxygen diffuses into red blood cells

Carbon dioxide diffuses into alveolus

Figure 19

Gas Exchange through the Alveolar Cell Sac

This figure depicts the exchange of oxygen and carbon dioxide in the lung alveolar sac in cross section. As air is pulled through the lung and into the small alveolar containing sacs by inhalation, oxygen gas seamlessly diffuses through alveolar and capillary cells and then into awaiting red blood cells in the capillary lumen. At the same time, carbon dioxide gas is released by red blood cells and diffuses the other way, through the capillary and then alveolar cell to be pushed out of the lung with expiration. The volume of gas exchange becomes dependent on the rate and force of air movement into and out of the alveolar sac, the blood and red cell volume flowing to the sac, the surface area exposure of capillary- and alveolar-cell outer membranes and the amount of chronic inflammation accrued on the outer-membrane surfaces and interstitial space between alveolar and capillary cells. The volume of interstitial space inflammation and the venues it is associated with, such as chronic scarring, blunts the exchange of gases.

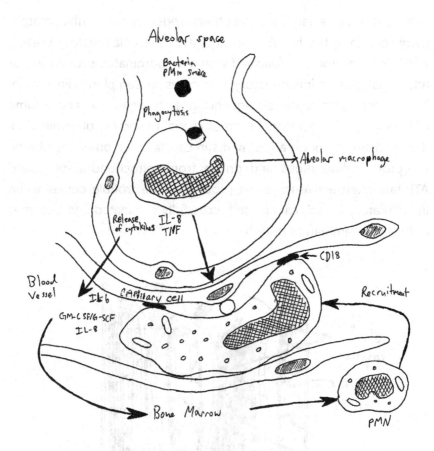

Alveolar space

Bacteria
PM10 Smoke

Phagocytosis

Alveolar macrophage

Release
of cytokines IL-8
TNF

CD18

Blood
Vessel

IL-6 Capillary cell

Recruitment

GM-CSF/G-SCF
IL-8

Bone Marrow

PMN

Figure 20

The Recruitment of the Immune Arsenal to Plume Inflammation and Combat Acute Breach in the Alveolar Space

Regardless of what foreign matter (bacteria, virus, particulate, noxious gas from the inhaled air) enters the alveolar space the alveolar cell will, in combination with alveolar macrophages, signal the adjoining capillary cell(s) within the alveolar sac to provide an inflammatory response from blood plasma to match the inflammatory breach. This causes capillary-cell outer membranes to increase their permeability to elicit a specific inflammatory mediator response to eliminate it. In the figure, this response includes different cytokines, IL-6, IL-8, TNF (tumor necrosis factor), and PMNs (neutrophil white blood cells), but could certainly involve others. Together, these inflammatory mediators form the initial containment of the inflammatory breach, which is then promptly followed with the coordinated sequencing of additional sets of inflammatory mediators to complete elimination. The proper coordination of sequencing, as to type, rate, and volume of inflammatory mediators becomes crucial to successful elimination. It is mediated through adjustments in capillary-cell outer-membrane receptor configurations and driven from mitochondrial-produced ATP-facilitated active-transport processes. The trouble comes when inflammatory breach cannot be successfully eliminated and becomes a chronic inflammatory breach.

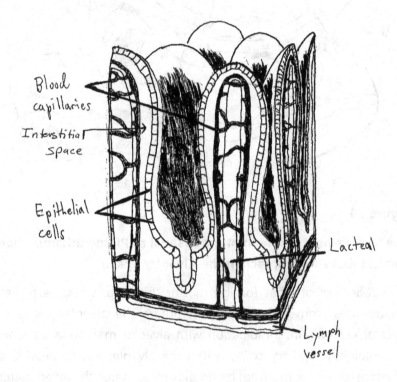

Figure 21

Intestinal Absorption of Nutrients

Capillary cells throughout the intestinal tract cohabitate with epithelial cells within intestinal crypts to facilitate absorption of nutrient, water and electrolytes. Absorption of nutrients becomes dependent on the quality of nutrients ingested, which directly affects the quality of intestinal microbiome. Foods with more plant fiber improve the quality of bacteria in the microbiome and cause a more complete absorption of carbohydrates, proteins, and antioxidants. Chronic ingestion of refined sugars and saturated animal fats, changes the type of bacteria contained within the intestinal microbiome. The result is reduced absorption of valuable nutrient and excessive surges of sugar through the intestinal crypts and into the portal vein circulation, which then is transported to the liver sinusoid. The sugar surge, especially if repeated over time, increases blood sugars, AGEs, LDL cholesterol and triglycerides to increase biases towards chronic interstitial space inflammation everywhere. Chronic intestinal interstitial-space inflammation caused by highly refined nutrient increases "leaky gut" syndrome, preventing quality nutrient from being absorbed and more toxic proinflammatory nutrient to pass into the portal vein to the liver.

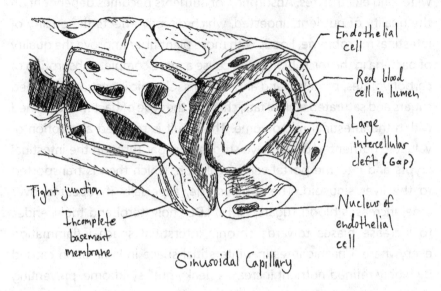

Labels on figure:
- Endothelial cell
- Red blood cell in lumen
- Large intercellular cleft (Gap)
- Nucleus of endothelial cell
- Tight junction
- Incomplete basement membrane

Sinusoidal Capillary

Figure 22

Sinusoidal Capillary Cell

This figure demonstrates in three dimensions how capillary cells in the liver have modified their outer membranes to accommodate maximum exposure of blood plasma to liver hepatocytes. The capillary-cell outer membrane framework in the liver sinusoid is loose, with gaps (incomplete) in their basement membranes and large intercellular clefts (spaces). All of these outer-membrane adjustments allow backwash of most blood plasma constituents onto liver cells in the sinusoid. This makes the liver hepatocyte vulnerable to inflammatory content within the blood plasma but also enables the liver cell to have rapid and direct access to portal vein nutrient without having to go through much access bureaucracy from the capillary cell. Because of this direct exposure to blood plasma, the liver becomes at for metastatic seeding of cancer cells and infectious agents that are traveling within the blood plasma.

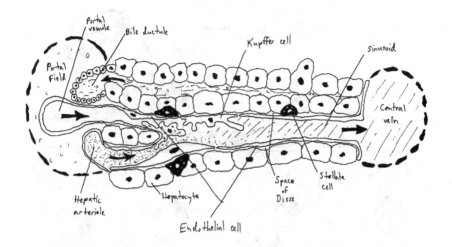

Figure 23

A Liver Sinusoid

In this depiction, blood flows left to right, whereas bile flow is from right to left. As portal vein and artery blood comingle and enter the sinusoid, it is met by a unique set of loosely arranged capillary cells whose outer membranes contain many pores, fenestra and gaps. This allows for a quicker dispersal of blood plasma constituents to enter the space of Disse (the interstitial space of the liver sinusoid). Imbedded within the interstitial space of Disse and lying close to capillary cells are specialized mesenchymal cells (or helper cells) known as Kupffer cells. Together with other mesenchymal cells, including stellate cells, they have become an accessory arm to the capillary-cell outer membranes patrol in protecting the vulnerable hepatocytes from potentially toxic blood plasma exposures. Stellate cells are specialized pericytes that can also store fat, but with chronic liver inflammation within the space of Disse, secrete an amyloid substance to increase scarring (fibrosis, cirrhosis). The amyloid goo, which is similar to that secreted by mesenchymal cells in the blood brain barrier in response to chronic inflammation, signals declines in liver cell function and the likely progression to cirrhosis of the liver.

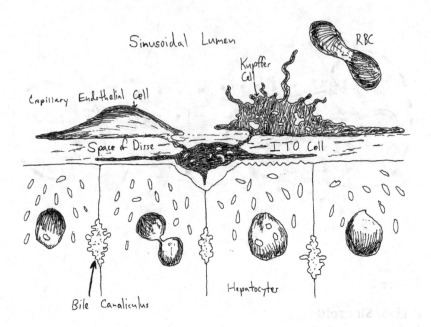

Figure 24

Close-Up View—Liver Sinusoid

In this figure, hepatocytes are at the bottom of the illustration and capillary cells are at the top. A red blood cell is seen in the capillary-sinusoidal lumen. Almost appearing connected within the space of Disse are capillary cells abutted up against flat and sprawling Kupffer cells. Kupffer cells are specialized mesenchymal cells that provide an extra layer of quality assurance to space of Disse immune surveillance. Along with stellate cells, the Kupffer cells couple with capillaries to form a dynamic trio that protects and the space of Disse from unwanted invaders. Although under entirely different context, this trio functions similarly in providing immune surveillance to protect liver cells as the astrocyte-pericyte and capillary cell complex that forms the blood brain barrier and protects brain nerve cells.

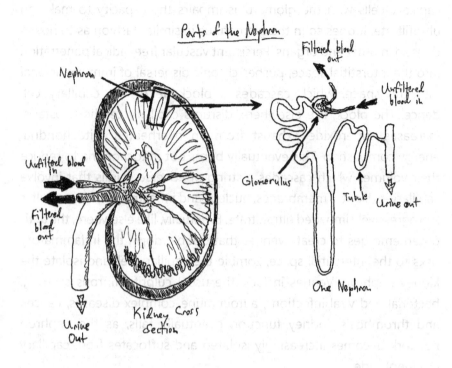

Parts of the Nephron

Nephron

Filtered blood out

Unfiltered blood in

Unfiltered blood in

Filtered blood out

Glomerulus

Tubule

Urine out

Urine Out

Kidney Cross Section

One Nephron

Figure 25

The Kidney Nephron

The adult kidney is made up of one million nephrons, which are the small filtering units that produce urine. Filtering is required to remove toxic waste from blood plasma that would otherwise interfere with functioning of other end organs. The most important part of the nephron is the glomerulus, where podocytes and capillary cells come together in Bowman's capsule to cause initial filtering of blood plasma. The initial filtered liquid is called an ultrafiltrate. The ultrafiltrate eventually leaves the glomerulus, and passes into a series of long tubes known as convoluted tubules. In these tubules, adjustments are made in the ultrafiltrate to the concentration of electrolytes and minerals. After completing the migration through the convoluted tubules, the ultrafiltrate has now become urine and is subsequently passed down a large tube from the kidney and collected in a sac known as a bladder. Chronic inflammation in the interstitial space between podocyte and capillary cells with the glomerulus impairs the capacity to make an ultrafiltrate. It does so in the glomerulus in similar fashion as to how it does so in other end organs. Persistent vascular free radical penetration into the interstitial space, pushes chronic dispersal of immune arsenal into the space, which cascades a blockade of the capillary cell dance. The block, like elsewhere, disrupts capillary cell homeostasis, increases superoxide exhaust from an overheated mitochondrial energy combustion. This eventually burns out mitochondria to reduce their volumes which cascades a string of adverse spirals that involve capillary-cell outer membranes, nucleus and infrastructure. The result is a progressively impaired ultrafiltrate. Eventually, like elsewhere, the anti-organ emerges to create venues that double down the inflammatory risks to the interstitial space, zombie the capillary cell and isolate the kidney nephron. Venues include the usual culprits, fibrous scarring, bacterial and viral infections, autoimmune-complex diseases, cancer, and thrombosis. Kidney function eventually fails, as the nephron network becomes increasingly isolated and suffocates from capillary cell ineptitude.

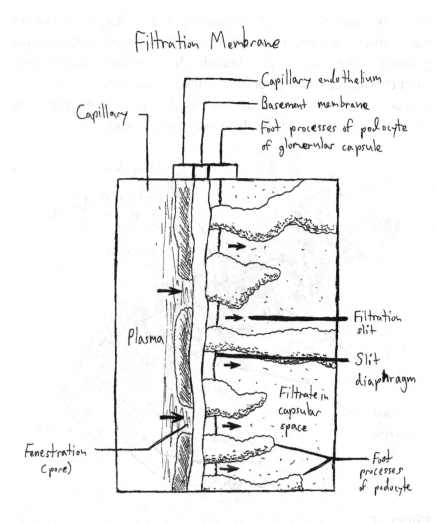

Figure 26

Cross Section—Capillary and Podocyte Cell

Blood plasma enters the kidney glomerulus (left of the figure), the first part of a nephron where ultrafiltrate is produced. The figure depicts a capillary cell with pores, a continuous basement membrane, and specialized filtering diaphragms. Opposite the capillary-cell basement membrane and across the narrow interstitial space, is the amoeba-like podocyte cell with multiple foot (pod) processes that abut the capillary cell basement membrane. The presence of pods increases the filtering surface area that is exposed to the capillary cell basement membrane. When blood plasma filtering has been completed within the glomerulus, the resulting ultrafiltrate has had the lion's share of waste product removed. With chronic interstitial-space inflammation in the glomerulus more filtering mistakes are made, and the interstitial space becomes increasingly vulnerable to anti-organ venues.

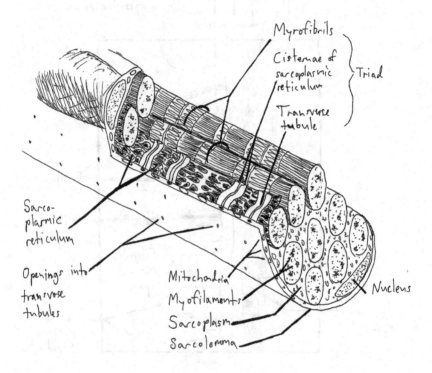

Figure 27

Cross Section—Skeletal Muscle

Skeletal muscle cells are composed of sliding actin-myosin filaments which are encapsulated by an outer membrane known as a sarcolemma. Next to the sarcolemma are densely packed mitochondria. Adjacent to the muscle cell, lying across a narrow interstitial space but not depicted in the figure, are capillary cells, which support large fluctuations to on-demand oxygen and nutrient (energy substrate) based on how fast and with how much force actin myosin filaments are sliding. In dramatic contrast to capillary cell mitochondria, which supply only

10% of all capillary cell energy, mitochondria of skeletal muscle supply 90 percent of all the energy that actin-myosin filament sliding utilizes. Therefore the volume of mitochondria within skeletal muscle is in direct proportion to how much exercise the skeletal muscle is performing. Whereas actin- myosin filament thickness determines force of sliding and skeletal muscle power, the presence of a dense mitochondrial network within muscle cells determines its endurance. The capability of skeletal muscle to perform optimally is based on regular use and the capability of capillary cells to prevent the interstitial space from becoming chronically inflamed. Preventing chronic inflammation within interstitial spaces of skeletal muscle cells becomes dependent on the volume and persistence of vascular inflammatory free radicals that are circulating in the blood. Preventing chronic inflammation in the interstitial space is mandatory if skeletal muscle is to perform optimally and not atrophy (sarcopenia). It hinges on the capacity of capillary cells to flux dance the permeability pivot and combustion pendulum swing.

Bibliography

Abbott, N. J., L. Ronnback, and E. Hansson. "Astrocyte-endothelial interactions at the blood-brain barrier." *Nature Reviews Neuroscience* (2006) 7:41–53.

Afanas'EV, I. B. "Mechanism of superoxide-mediated damage relevance to mitochondrial aging." *Annals of the New York Academy of Sciences* (2004) 1019: 260–64.

Ahmadi, N., F. Hajsadeghi, K. Gul, J. Vane, N. Usman, F. Flores, K. Nasir, H. Hecht, M. Naghavi, and M. Budoff. "Relations between digital thermal monitoring of vascular function, the Framingham risk score and coronary calcium score." *Journal of Cardiovascular Computed Tomography* (2008) 2: 382–88.

Aliev, G., H. H. Palacios, E. Gasimov, M. E. Obrenovich, L. Moralis, J. Leszek, V. Bragin, A. S. Herrera, and D. Gokhman. "Oxidative stress-induced mitochondrial failure and vascular hypoperfusion as a key initiator for the development of Alzheimer's disease." *Pharmaceuticals* (2010) 3 (1): 158–87.

Aliev, G., D. Sevidova, B. T. Lamb, M. E. Obrenovich, S. L. Siedlak, H. V. Vinters, R. P. Friedland, J. C. Lamanna, M. A. Smith, and G. Perry. "Mitochondria and vascular lesions as a central target for the development of Alzheimer's disease and Alzheimer's disease-like pathology in transgenic mice." *Neurological Research* (2003) 25 (6): 665–74.

Aliev, G., D. Seyidova, M. L. Neal, J. Shi, B. T. Lamb, S. L. Siedlak, H. V. Vinters, E. Head, G. Perry, J. C. Lamanna, R. P. Friedland, and C. W. Cotman. "Atherosclerosis lesions and mitochondria DNA deletions in brain microvessels as a central target for the development of human AD and AD-like pathology in aged transgenic mice." *Annals of the New York Academy of Sciences* (2002) 977: 45–64.

Aliev, G., M. A. Smith, M. E. Obrenovich, J. de la Torre, and G. Perry. "Role of vascular hypoperfusion-induced oxidative stress and mitochondrial failure in the pathogenesis of Alzheimer's disease." *Neurotoxicity Research* (2003) 5 (7):491–504.

Ames, B. N. "Low micronutrient intake may accelerate the degenerative diseases of aging through allocation of scarce micronutrients by triage." *Proceedings of the National Academy of Sciences of the United States of America* 103 (47): 17589–94.

Ames, B. N., H. Atamna, and D. W. Kililea. "Mineral and vitamin deficiencies can accelerate the mitochondrial decay of aging." *Molecular Aspects of Medicine* 26 (4–5): 363–78.

Atamna, H. "Heme, iron and the mitochondrial decay of ageing." *Ageing Research Reviews* (2004) 3 (3): 303–18.

Ballinger, S. W. "Mitochondrial dysfunction in cardiovascular disease." *Free Radical Biology and Medicine* (2005) 38 (10): 1278–95.

Barja, G., and A. Herrero. "Oxidative damage to mitochondrial DNA is inversely related to maximum life span in the heart and brain of mammals." *FASEB Journal* (2000) 14 (2): 312–18.

Benoit, V., G. Bruno, N. Sanz-Garcia, J. Leclerc, M. Foretz, and A. Fabrizio. "Cellular and molecular mechanisms of metformin: an overview." *Clinical Science (London)* 122 (6): 25370.

Berneburg, M., Y. Kamenisch, and J. Krutmann. "Repair of mitochondrial DNA in aging and carcinogenesis." *Photochemical and Photobiological Sciences* (2006) (5): 190–98.

Brownlee, M. "The pathobiology of diabetic complications, a unifying mechanism." *Diabetes* (2005) 64 (6): 1615–25.

Buckingham, Robert. *Hazing Aging: How Capillary Endothelia Control Inflammation and Aging.* Bloomington, IN: iUniverse, 2015.

Bullon, P., H. N. Newman, and M. Battino. "Obesity, diabetes mellitus, atherosclerosis and chronic periodontitis: a shared pathology via oxidative stress and mitochondrial dysfunction." *Periodontology* (2014) 64 (1): 139–53.

Church, T. S., J. L. Kuk, R. Ross, E. L. Priest, E. Biltoff, and S. N. Blair. "Association of cardiorespiratory fitness, body mass index, and waist circumference to nonalcoholic fatty liver disease." *Gastroenterology* (2006) 130: 2023–30.

Circu, M. L., and T. Y. Aw. "Reactive oxygen species, cellular redox systems and apoptosis." *Free Radical Biology and Medicine* (2010) 48 (6): 749–62.

Dai, D. F., P. S. Rabinovitch, and Z. Ungvari. "Mitochondria and cardiovascular aging." *Circulation Research* (2012) 110: 1109–24.

Davidson, S. M., and M. R. Duchen. "Endothelial mitochondria contributing to vascular function and disease." *Circulation Research* 100: 1128–41.

De la Torre, J. C. "Is Alzheimer's disease a neurodegenerative or vascular disorder? Data, dogma and dialectics." *Lancet Neurology* (2004) 3 (3):184–90.

Deichmann, R., C. Lavie, and S. Andrews "Coenzyme Q_{10} and statin-induced mitochondrial dysfunction." *Ochsner Journal* 10 (1): 16–21.

Demaurex, N., D. Poburko, and M. Frieden. "Regulation of plasma membrane calcium fluxes by mitochondria." *Biochimica et Biophysica Acta (BBA)—Bioenergetics* 1787 (11): 1383–94.

Depeint, F., W. R. Bruce, N. Shangari, R. Mehta, and P. J. O'Brien. "Mitochondrial function and toxicity: role of B vitamins in the one carbon transfer pathways." *Chemico-Biological Interactions* 163 (1–2): 113–32.

Di Lisa, F., N. Kaludercic, A. Carpi, R. Menabo, and M. Gorgio. "Mitochondria and vascular pathology." *Pharmacology Reports* (2009) 61 (1): 123–30.

Doughan, A. K., D. G. Harrison, and S. I. Dikalov. "Molecular mechanisms of angiotensin II-mediated mitochondrial dysfunction, linking mitochondrial oxidative damage and vascular endothelial dysfunction." *Circulation Research* (2008) 102: 488–96.

Droge, W. "Free radicals in the physiological controls of cell function." *Physiological Reviews* (2002) 82 (1): 47–95.

Dromparis, P., and E. D. Michelakis. "Mitochondria in vascular health and disease." *Annual Review of Physiology* (2013) 75: 95–126.

Duchen, M. R. "Role of mitochondria in health and disease." *Diabetes* (2004) 53 suppl. 1: S96–S102.

Duda, M. K., K. M. O'Shea, and W. C. Stanley. "Omega-3 polyunsaturated fatty acid supplementation for the treatment of heart failure: mechanisms and clinical potential." *Cardiovascular Research* 84: 33–41.

Dumon, M., K. Kipiani, F. Yu, E. Wille, M. Katz, N. Y. Calingasan, G. K. Gouras, M. T. Lin, and M. F. Beal. "Coenzyme Q_{10} decreases amyloid pathology and improves behavior in a transgenic mouse model of Alzheimer's disease." *Journal of Alzheimer's Disease* (2011) 27 (1): 211–23.

Durante, L. "Mitochondria—a nexus for aging, calorie restriction, and sirtuins." *Cell* (2008) 132 (2): 171–76.

Erusalimsky, J. D., and S. Moncada. "Nitric oxide and mitochondrial signaling, from physiology to pathophysiology." *Arteriosclerosis, Thrombosis, and Vascular Pathology* (2007) 27: 2524–53.

Esposito, L., J. Raber, L. Kekonius, F. Yan, G. Q. Yu, N. Bien-Ly, J. Puolivali, K. Scearce-Levie, E. Masliah, and L. Mucke. "Reduction in mitochondrial superoxide dismutase modulates Alzheimer's disease-like pathology and accelerates the onset of behavioral changes in human amyloid precursor protein transgenic mice." *Journal of Neuroscience* (2006) 26 (19): 5167–79.

Ferretta, A., A. Gaballo, P. Tanzarella, C. Piccoli, N. Capitanio, B. Nico, T. Annese, M. Di Paola, C. Dell'Aquila, M. De Mari, E. Ferranini, V. Bonifati, C. Pacelli, and T. Cocco. "Effect of resveratrol on mitochondrial function: implications in parkin-associated familiar Parkinson's disease." *Biochimica et Biophysica Acta (BBA)—Molecular Basis of Disease* (2014) 1842 (7): 902–15.

Folli, F., D. Corradi, P. Fanti, A. Davalli, A. Paez, A. Giaccari, C. Perego, and G. Muscogiuri. "The role of oxidative stress in the pathogenesis of type 2 diabetes mellitus micro and macrovascular complication: avenues for a mechanistic-based therapeutic approach." *Current Diabetes Reviews* (2011) 7 (5): 313–24.

Forstermann, U. "Oxidative stress in vascular disease: causes, defense mechanisms and potential therapies." *Nature Reviews Cardiology* (2008) 5: 338–49.

Giacco, F., and M. Brownlee. "Oxidative stress and diabetic complications." *Circulation Research* (2010) 107: 1058–70.

Gutierrez, J., S. W. Ballinger, V. M. Darley-Usmar, and A. Landar. "Free radicals, mitochondria, and oxidized lipids, the emerging role in signal transduction in vascular cells." *Circulation Research* (2006) 99: 924–32.

Hamburg, N. M., M. J. Keyes, M. G. Larson, R. S. Vasan, R. Schnabel, M. M. Pryde, G. F. Mitchell, J. Sheffy, J. A. Vita, and E. J. Benjamin. "Cross-sectional relations of digital vascular function to cardiovascular risk factors in the Framingham Heart Study." *Circulation* (2008) 117: 2467–74.

Haraldsson, B. S. "The endothelium as part of the integrative glomerular barrier complex. *Kidney International* 85 (1): 8–11.

Hawkins, B. T., and T. P. David. "The blood-brain barrier/neurovascular unit in health and disease." *Pharmacological Reviews* 57 (2): 173–85.

Johnson, N. A., T. Sachinwalla, D. W. Walton, K. Smith, A. Armstrong, M. W. Thompson, and J. George. "Aerobic exercise training reduces hepatic and visceral lipids in obese individuals without weight loss." *Hepatology* (2009) 50 (4): 1105–12.

Knowler, W. C., E. Barrett-Connor, S. E. Fowler, R. F. Hamman, J. M. Lachin, and E. A. Walker. "Reduction in the incidence of type 2 diabetes with lifestyle intervention or metformin." *New England Journal of Medicine* (2002) 346: 393–403.

Li, X., P. Fang, J. Mai, E. T. Choi, H. Wang, and X. F. Yang. "Targeting mitochondria reactive oxygen species as novel therapy for inflammatory diseases and cancers." *Journal of Hematology and Oncology* 6 (19): 1756–1872.

Liang, H., and W. F. Ward. "PGC-1-alpha: a key regulator of energy metabolism." *Advances in Physiology Education* 30 (4): 145–51.

Lidz, F. "Alpha is the name, baseball is the game, and obsession is the result." *Sports Illustrated* (December 1980).

Lin, C. J., T. H. Chen, L. Y. Yang, and C. M. Shih. "Resveratrol protects astrocytes against traumatic brain injury through inhibiting apoptotic and autophagic cell death." *Cell Death and Disease* (2014) 5: e1147.

Lin, M. T., and M. F. Beal. "Mitochondrial dysfunction and oxidative stress in neurodegenerative diseases." *Nature* (2006) 443 (7113): 787–95.

Littarru, G. P., and L. Tiano. "Bioenergetic and antioxidant properties of coenzyme Q_{10}: recent developments." *Molecular Biotechnology* 37 (1): 31–37.

Liu, T. F., and C. E. McCall. "Deacetylation of sirt 1 reprograms inflammation and cancer." *Journal of Clinical Investigation* (2010) 120 (7): 2267–70.

Madamanchi, N. R., and M. S. Runge. "Mitochondrial dysfunction in atherosclerosis." *Circulation Research* (2007) 100: 460–73.

Madamanchi, N. R., A. Vendrov, and M. S. Runge. "Oxidative stress and vascular disease." *Arteriosclerosis, Thrombosis and Vascular Disease* (2005) 25: 29–38.

Mathews, D. C., M. Davies, J. Murray, S. Williams, W. H. Tsui, Y. Li, R. D. Andrews, A. Lukic, P. McHugh, S. Vallabhajosula, M. J. de Leon, and L. Mosconi. "Physical activity, Mediterranean diet and biomarkers—assessed risk for Alzheimer's disease: a multi-modality brain imaging study." *Advanced Molecular Imaging* (2014) 4 (4): 43–57.

Matsuda, M., and I. Shimomura. "Increased oxidative stress in obesity: implications for metabolic syndrome, diabetes, hypertension, dyslipidemia, atherosclerosis, and cancer." *Obesity Research & Clinical Practice* (2013) 7 (3): e330–e341.

Mattagajasingh, I., C. S. Kim, A. Naqvi, T. Yamamori, T. A. Hoffman, S. B. Jung, J. DeRicco, K. Kasuno, and K. Irani. "SIRT 1 promotes endothelium-dependent vascular relaxation by activating endothelial nitric oxide synthetase." *Proceedings of the National Academy of Sciences of the United States of America* (2007) 104 (37): 14855–60.

Melitis, C. D., and K. Wilkes. "Mitochondria: overlooking these small organelles can have huge clinical consequences in treating virtually every disease." *Townsend Letter* (2015) 383: 50–56.

Miller, R. A., and M. J. Birnbaum. "An energetic tale of AMPK-independent effects of metformin." *Journal of Clinical Investigation* (2010) 120 (7): 2267–70.

Mitchell, Y., and V. Darley-Usmar. "Metabolic syndrome and mitochondrial dysfunction: insights from preclinical studies with a mitochondrially targeted antioxidant." *Free Radical Biology and Medicine* (2012) 52 (5): 838–40.

Mosconi, L., J. Murray, M. Davies, S. Williams, E. Pirraglia, N. Spector, W. H. Tsui, Y. Li, T. Butler, R. S. Osorio, L. Glodzik, S. Vallabhajosular, P. McHugn, C. R. Marmar, and M. J. de Leon. "Nutrient intake and brain biomarkers of Alzheimer's disease in at-risk cognitively normal individuals: a cross-sectional neuroimaging pilot study." *BMJ Open* (2014) 4 (6): e004850.

Mueller, C. F. H., K. Laude, J. S. McNally, and D. G. Harrison. "Redox mechanisms in blood vessels." *Arteriosclerosis, Thrombosis, and Vascular Biology* (2005) 25: 274–78.

Munzel, T., T. Gori, R. M. Bruno, and S. Taddei. "Is oxidative stress a therapeutic target in cardiovascular disease?" *European Heart Journal* (2010) 396: 2741–48.

Nakagami, H., Y. Kaneda, T. Ogihara, and R. Morishita. "Endothelial dysfunction in hyperglycemia as a trigger of atherosclerosis." *Current Diabetes Reviews* (2005) 1 (1): 59–63.

Nicolson, G. L. "Mitochondrial dysfunction and chronic disease: treatment with natural supplements." *Alternative Therapies in Health and Medicine* (2014) 15: 40–51.

Pagano, G., A. A. Talamanca, G. Castello, M. D. Cordero, M. d'Ischia, M. N. Gadaleta, F. V. Pallardo, S. Petrovic, L. Tiano, and A. Zatterale. "Oxidative stress and mitochondrial dysfunction across broad-ranging pathologies: toward mitochondria-targeted clinical strategies." *Oxidative Medicine Cellular Longevity* (2014): 541230.

Patel, S. P., P. G. Sullivan, J. D. Pandya, G. A. Goldstein, J. L. VanRooyen, H. M. Yonutas, K. C. Eldahan, J. Morehouse, D. S. K. Magnuson, and A. G. Rabchevsky. "N-acetyl cysteine amide preserves mitochondrial bioenergetics and improves functional recovery following spinal trauma." *Experimental Neurology* (2014) 257: 95–105.

Pieczenik, S. R., and J. Neustadt. "Mitochondrial dysfunction and molecular pathways of disease." *Experimental and Molecular Pathology* (2007) 83 (1): 84–92.

Qiu, X., K. Brown, M. D. Hirschey, E. Verdin, and D. Chen. "Calorie restriction reduces oxidative stress by SIRT 3-mediated activation." *Cell Metabolism* (2010) 12 (6): 662–67.

Radaelli, R., C. E. Botton, E. N. Wihelm, M. Bottaro, F. Lacerda, A. Gaya, K. Moraes, A. Peruzzolo, L. E. Brown, and R. S. Pinto. "Low- and high-volume strength training induces similar neuromuscular improvements in muscle quality in elderly women." *Experimental Gerontology* (2013) 48 (8): 710–16.

Rafnsson, S. B., V. Dilis, and A. Trichopoulou. "Antioxidant nutrients and age-related cognitive decline: a systematic review of population-based cohort studies. *European Journal of Nutrition* (2013) 52 (6): 1553–67.

Ramachandran, A., A. L. Levonen, P. S. Brookes, E. Ceaser, S. Shiva, M. C. Barone, and V. Darley-Usmar. "Mitochondria, nitric oxide and cardiovascular dysfunction." *Free Radical Biology and Medicine* (2002) 33 (11): 1465–74.

Rask-Madsen, C., and G. L. King. "Mechanisms of disease: endothelial dysfunction in insulin resistance and diabetes." *Nature Reviews Endocrinology* (2007) 3: 46–56.

Reddy, P. H., and M. F. Beal. "Are mitochondria critical in the pathogenesis of Alzheimer's disease?" *Brain Research Review* (2005) 49 (3): 618–32.

Reeve, A. K., K. J. Krishnan, and D. M. Turnbull. "Age-related mitochondrial degenerative disorders in humans." *Biotechnology Journal* (2008) 3 (6): 750–56.

Rizos, E. C., E. E. Ntzani, E. Bika, M. S. Kostapanos, and M. S. Elisaf. "Association between omega-3 fatty acid supplementation and major risk of cardiovascular disease events: a systematic review and meta-analysis." *Journal of the American Medical Association* (2012) 308: 1024–33.

Schonfeld, P., and G. Reise. "Why does brain metabolism not favor burning fatty acids to provide energy?—Reflections on disadvantages of the use of free fatty acids as fuel for brain." *Journal of Cerebral Blood Flow and Metabolism* 33: 1493–99.

Semenza, G. L. "Oxygen sensing, homeostasis and disease." *New England Journal of Medicine* (2011) 365: 537–47.

Shen, G. X. "Oxidative stress and diabetic cardiovascular disorders: roles of mitochondria and NADPH oxidase." *Canadian Journal of Physiology and Pharmacology* (2010) 88 (3): 241–48.

Shojaee-Moradie, F., K. C. Baynes, C. Pentecost, J. D. Bell, E. L. Thomas, N. C. Jackson, M. Stolinski, M. Whyte, D. Lovell, S. B. Bowes, J. Gibney, R. H. Jones, and A. M. Umpleby. "Exercise training reduces fatty acid availability and improves the insulin sensitivity of glucose metabolism." *Diabetologia* (2007) 50: 404–13.

Singh, B., A. K. Parsaik, M. M. Mielke, P. J. Erwin, D. S. Knopman, R. C. Petersen, and R. O. Roberts. "Association of Mediterranean diet with mild cognitive impairment and Alzheimer's disease: a systematic review and meta-analysis." *Journal of Alzheimer's Disease* (2014) 39 (2): 271–82.

Singh, K. K. "Mitochondrial dysfunction is a common phenotype in aging and cancer." *Annals of the New York Academy of Sciences* (2004) 1019: 260–64.

Sprague, A. H., and R. A. Khalil. "Inflammatory cytokines in vascular dysfunction and vascular disease." *Biochemical Pharmacology* (2009) 78 (6): 539–52.

Svistounov, D., S. N. Zykova, V. C. Cogger, A. Warren, A. C. McMahan, R. Fraser, and D. G. Le Conteur. "Liver sinusoidal endothelial cells and regulation of blood lipoproteins." In *Dyslipidemia from Practice to Treatment*. Edited by Roya Kelishadi. INTECH Open Access Publisher (2012): 263–78.

Tang, X., Y. X. Luo, H. Z. Chen, and D. P. Liu. "Mitochondria, endothelial cell function and vascular diseases." *Frontiers in Physiology (2014)* dx.doi.org/10.3389, 00175.

Toren, F., and N. J. Holbrook. "Oxidants, oxidative stress and the biology of ageing." *Nature* (2000) 408: 239–47.

Valle, I., A. Alvarez-Barrientos, E. Arza, S. Lamas, and M. Monsalve. "PGC-1-alpha regulates the mitochondrial antioxidant defense system in vascular endothelial cells." *Cardiovascular Research* (2005) 66: 562–73.

Victor, V., N. Apostolova, R. Herance, A. Hernandez-Mijares, and M. Rocha. "Oxidative stress and mitochondrial dysfunction in atherosclerosis: mitochondrial-targeted antioxidants as potential therapy." *Current Medicinal Chemistry* (2009) 16 (53): 4654–67.

Viollet, B., and B. Foretz. "Revisiting the mechanisms of metformin action in the liver." *Annales d'Endocrinologie (Paris)* (2013) 74 (2): 123–29.

Viollet, B., B. Guigas, N. S. Garcia, J. Lelclerc, M. Foretz, and F. Andreeli. "Cellular and molecular mechanisms of metformin: an overview." *Clinical Science (London)* (2012) 122 (6): 253–70.

Wang, D. M., S. Q. Li, W. L. Wu, X. Y. Zhu, Y. Wang, and H. Y. Yuan. "Effects of long-term treatment with quercetin on cognition and mitochondrial function in the mouse model of Alzheimer's disease." *Neurochemical Research* (2014) 39 (8): 1533–43.

Wang, J. C., and M. Bennett. "Aging and atherosclerosis." *Circulation Research* (2012) 111: 245–59.

Wang, W. Y., M. S. Tan, and J. T. Tan. "Role of proinflammatory cytokines released from microglia in Alzheimer's disease." *Annals of Translational Medicine* (2015) 3 (10): 136.

Wong, R., C. Steenbergen, and E. Murphy. "Mitochondrial permeability transition pore and calcium handling." *Methods in Molecular Biology* 810: 235–42.

Yki-Jarvinen, H., "Fat in the liver and insulin resistance." *Annals of Medicine* (2005) 37: 347–56.

Yorek, M. A. "The role of oxidative stress in diabetic vascular and neural disease." *Free Radical Research* (2003) 37 (5): 471–80.

Yu, E., J. Mercer, and M. Bennett. "Mitochondria in vascular disease." *Cardiovascular Research* (2012) 95 (2): 173–82.

Zhu, X., M. A. Smith, K. Honda, G. Aliev, P. I. Moreira, A. Nunomura, G. Casadesus, P. L. R. Harris, S. L. Siedlak, and G. Perry. "Vascular oxidative stress in Alzheimer's disease vascular dementia—proceedings of the Fourth International Congress of Vascular Dementia." *Journal of Neurological Sciences* (2007) 257 (1–2): 240–46.

Zhu, Y., Y. Yan., D. R. Principe, X. Zou, A. Vassiloupos, and D. Gius. "SIRT 3 and SIRT 4 are mitochondrial tumor suppressor proteins that connect mitochondrial metabolism and carcinogenesis." *Cancer and Metabolism* (2014) 15 (2): 1–11.

Robert Buckingham, MD, FACP, is a practicing physician in private practice in Ojai, California. He received his medical and master's degrees from the University of Illinois in Chicago and received further training in medicine at Northwestern University in Chicago. He was elected as a Fellow in the American College of Physicians in 2009. He is also the author Hazing Aging, which was a runner-up book of the year in the health division from Forward Reviews. He remains passionate about practicing medicine and exploring the science of aging.

Index

arteriosclerosis/atherosclerosis 298, 299, 301, 303, 304, 305, 308, 309

arthritis pain 109, 132, 146

aspirin 50, 115, 146, 156, 157, 158, 159, 161, 177, 184, 187

asthma 26, 133, 144, 154, 164, 215

astrocytes 43, 46, 212, 226, 281, 303, *See also* glial cells

ATP (adenosine triphosphate) 66, 67, 69, 74, 75, 82, 83, 93, 179, 205, 206, 207, 218, 221, 222, 224, 228, 230, 232, 233, 234, 245, 266, 268, 271, 283, 286

autoimmune diseases 47, 110, 138, 151, 164, 202

axons 42, 44

B

B_1 (thiamine) 184, 185

B_2 (riboflavin) 184

B_3 (niacin) 51, 150, 151, 152, 153, 154, 174, 184, 185, 229, 239, 240

B_5 (pantothenic acid) 184

B_6 (pyridoxine) 184, 185, 229, *See also* vitamin B6

B_9 (folic acid) 183, 184, 185, 209

B_{12} (cobalamin) 124, 164, 184, 209

baby aspirin 156, 157, 184, 187

bacteria 32, 33, 35, 37, 66, 115, 124, 137, 164, 205, 233, 236, 244, 285, 287

basement membrane xix, 4, 17, 24, 39, 43, 44, 52, 76, 95, 97, 102, 111, 112, 118, 119, 149, 150,

151, 155, 157, 205, 212, 242, 244, 282, 293, 294

B complex vitamins/B vitamins 164, 183, 184, 185, 300

beans (as protein) 139, 142

behavioral changes/ modifications 301

beta-blockers 115, 161, 211, 212

blood-brain barrier 38, 212, 215, 221, 225, 226, 254, 280, 281, 282, 297, 302

blood clotting 38

blood pressure 41, 57, 122, 131, 138, 143, 151, 159, 160, 161, 162, 190, 207, 210, 211, 212, 213, 219, 230, 235

high blood pressure 159, 161, 162, 235, *See* high blood pressure

improvements in 3, 148, 306

increase 4, 7, 8, 15, 21, 22, 25, 28, 29, 30, 32, 33, 34, 38, 41, 42, 52, 53, 55, 57, 65, 69, 70, 72, 78, 84, 86, 93, 95, 98, 99, 101, 103, 104, 105, 109, 110, 112, 114, 117, 118, 129, 130, 131, 137, 138, 139, 143, 144, 145, 147, 148, 151, 153, 155, 157, 160, 162, 163, 164, 171, 174, 177, 178, 180, 186, 187, 205, 206, 207, 210, 212, 213, 216, 220, 223, 224, 225, 227, 228, 232, 233, 237, 238, 244, 245, 247, 249, 252,

C

lumens 4, 52, 95, 110, 119, 159, 160, 210, 222, 240, 247, 283

lungs 7, 14, 32, 49, 51, 131, 194, 222

lupus 262

M

macrophage 25, 285

magnesium 67, 68, 93, 94, 124, 178, 179, 180, 185, 214, 234

magnetic resonance imaging (MRI) scan 234

malabsorption 19, 34, 35, 233

maltose 28, 227

manganese 85, 172, 178, 181, 185, 214, 234, 275

Mediterranean diet 35, 157, 161, 175, 179, 183, 235, 304, 307

membrane morphology xix, xx, 24, 104

memory loss 44, 49, *See also* short-term memory loss

menopause 224, 246
    female 223, 246, 251
    male 251

mercury 139, 141, 142

metabolic syndrome 31, 136, 140, 220, 235, 252, 304

MET (metabolic equivalent) 123, 194, 196, 235, 253, 289

milk 140, 174, 196

MI (myocardial infarction) 53, 232, 238

ministroke 251

mitochondria xi, xiii, xviii, xx, 6, 9, 21, 22, 24, 25, 30, 40, 41, 42, 43, 46, 48, 50, 51, 52, 53, 55, 56, 57, 58, 61, 64, 65, 66, 67, 68, 69, 70, 71, 72, 74, 75, 78, 80, 81, 82, 83, 88, 90, 91, 92, 93, 94, 96, 97, 98, 101, 102, 104, 105, 127, 129, 130, 147, 149, 154, 158, 163, 166, 167, 168, 171, 172, 173, 174, 178, 179, 180, 182, 185, 200, 202, 205, 206, 207, 212, 213, 214, 215, 219, 222, 223, 224, 225, 226, 227, 236, 237, 238, 240, 242, 245, 247, 248, 253, 262, 264, 265, 269, 272, 273, 274, 276, 279, 282, 283, 292, 294, 295, 297, 298, 299, 300, 301, 302, 303, 304, 305, 306, 307, 308, 309

monosaccharide 70, 227

monounsaturated fats/oils 72, 136, 139, 140, 216, 235, 238, 246

morphology xix, xx, 24, 104, 238

mortality 175, 263, *See also* cardiovascular mortality; vascular mortality

multiple sclerosis (MS) 47, 238, 262

muscle pain 154, 225, 238, 249

myalgia 238

myocardial infarction (MI) 53, 232, 238

N

N-acetyl cysteine (NAC) 181, 182, 218, 239, 305

napping 146

nephron 39, 226, 239, 291,
    292, 293
neurodegenerative decline/disease
    44, 243, 299, 303
niacin (B$_3$) 51, 150, 151, 152, 153,
    154, 174, 184, 185, 229,
    239, 240
nitric oxide (NO) xiii, xviii, xix, xx,
    xxi, 2, 6, 7, 8, 9, 11, 19, 20, 21,
    22, 24, 25, 27, 39, 41, 42, 43,
    45, 46, 47, 48, 50, 51, 52, 53,
    56, 57, 58, 60, 61, 62, 64, 65,
    66, 67, 68, 69, 70, 74, 75, 81,
    82, 83, 85, 86, 93, 94, 98, 99,
    101, 102, 105, 111, 114, 119,
    120, 122, 124, 125, 127, 128,
    129, 130, 137, 141, 145, 147,
    148, 149, 150, 151, 152, 155,
    158, 160, 165, 166, 167, 168,
    169, 170, 171, 172, 173, 174,
    183, 184, 185, 191, 192, 195,
    197, 198, 201, 202, 203, 206,
    211, 216, 219, 221, 225, 230,
    234, 236, 237, 238, 240, 243,
    245, 249, 251, 258, 259, 266,
    268, 273, 275, 276, 277, 280,
    282, 283, 301, 304, 306
nucleus (of cell) xviii, 42, 67, 90,
    104, 168, 215, 219, 226, 240,
    241, 242, 292, 300
nutrient/oxygen support 238
nuts 85, 136, 139, 140, 141, 142,
    176, 238

O

obesity xvii, 28, 30, 71, 134, 136,
    140, 151, 213, 219, 220,
    227, 232, 233, 235, 241, 252,
    299, 304
obstructive sleep apnea 143, 241
occlusion 17, 119, 156, 241
omega-3 fatty acids 140, 176,
    177, 242
omega-3 oils 139, 175, 176, 177,
    178, 218
omega-6 fatty acids/oils 242
oncotic pressure 242
organelles 42, 66, 67, 105, 109,
    128, 165, 168, 215, 219, 221,
    236, 242, 243, 265, 304
    defined xix, 29, 34, 83, 208,
        213, 219, 230, 236,
        244, 250
    mitochondria xi, xiii, xviii, xx,
        6, 9, 21, 22, 24, 25, 30,
        40, 41, 42, 43, 46, 48, 50,
        51, 52, 53, 55, 56, 57, 58,
        61, 64, 65, 66, 67, 68, 69,
        70, 71, 72, 74, 75, 78, 80,
        81, 82, 83, 88, 90, 91, 92,
        93, 94, 96, 97, 98, 101,
        102, 104, 105, 127, 129,
        130, 147, 149, 154, 158,
        163, 166, 167, 168, 171,
        172, 173, 174, 178, 179,
        180, 182, 185, 200, 202,
        205, 206, 207, 212, 213,
        214, 215, 219, 222, 223,
        224, 225, 226, 227, 236,

329

V

vascular dementia 309
vascular endothelium 49
vascular inflammation 14, 122,
    125, 126, 229, 244, 250, 251
  acute 80, 167, 253, 277, 285
  chronic xiii, xv, xvi, xvii, xviii,
      xix, xx, xxi, xxii, 1, 2, 3,
      4, 5, 6, 7, 8, 9, 10, 11, 12,
      14, 15, 16, 17, 18, 19, 20,
      21, 22, 23, 24, 25, 26, 27,
      28, 29, 30, 31, 32, 33, 34,
      35, 37, 38, 40, 41, 44, 45,
      46, 47, 48, 49, 51, 52, 53,
      54, 55, 56, 57, 58, 59, 60,
      61, 62, 63, 64, 66, 72, 75,
      76, 79, 80, 81, 84, 85, 86,
      87, 88, 89, 90, 91, 92, 93,
      95, 96, 98, 99, 100, 101,
      103, 104, 105, 106, 108,
      109, 110, 111, 112, 113,
      114, 115, 116, 117, 119,
      120, 121, 122, 123, 125,
      126, 127, 128, 129, 131,
      133, 134, 135, 137, 138,
      140, 141, 142, 143, 144,
      145, 146, 147, 148, 149,
      150, 151, 152, 154, 155,
      156, 157, 158, 159, 160,
      161, 162, 163, 164, 165,
      167, 169, 170, 171, 173,
      176, 178, 179, 180, 182,
      183, 185, 186, 187, 188,
      189, 197, 198, 199, 200,
      201, 202, 203, 204, 205,
      206, 207, 209, 211, 215,
      216, 218, 220, 225, 226,
      227, 230, 233, 235, 237,
      240, 241, 243, 244, 247,
      248, 249, 250, 251, 254,
      257, 258, 259, 260, 261,
      262, 263, 272, 274, 277,
      281, 283, 284, 286, 287,
      289, 291, 292, 294, 295,
      299, 305
  impact of 51
vascular inflammatory risk factors
    4, 263
vascular tree 12, 18, 98, 118, 197,
    210, 223
vasoactive endothelial growth
    factor (VEGF) 95, 253
vasoconstriction/vasoconstrictors
    159, 160
vegetables 34, 35, 138, 139, 141,
    142, 186, 187, 203, 235
very low density (VLDL)
    cholesterol 253
vision 219, *See also* eyes
vitamin C 182
vitamin D$_3$ 169, 170
vitamin D deficiency 168, 169,
    170, 245
vitamin D supplementation 170
vitamin E 181, 182
vitamin K2 169, 170, 171
vitamins and supplements, *See
    also specific vitamins and
    supplements*
  B complex vitamins 183,
      184, 185

330

TRUE DIRECTIONS
An affiliate of Tarcher Perigee

OUR MISSION

Tarcher Perigee's mission has always been to publish
books that contain great ideas. Why? Because:

GREAT LIVES BEGIN WITH GREAT IDEAS

At Tarcher Perigee, we recognize that many talented authors, speakers,
educators, and thought-leaders share this mission and deserve to be published –
many more than Tarcher Perigee can reasonably publish ourselves. True
Directions is ideal for authors and books that increase awareness, raise
consciousness, and inspire others to live their ideals and passions.

Like Tarcher Perigee, True Directions books are designed to do three things:
inspire, inform, and motivate.

Thus, True Directions is an ideal way for these important voices to
bring their messages of hope, healing, and help to the world.

Every book published by True Directions– whether it is non-fiction, memoir,
novel, poetry or children's book – continues Tarcher Perigee's mission to publish
works that bring positive change in the world. We invite you to join our mission.

For more information, see the True Directions website:

www.iUniverse.com/TrueDirections/SignUp

Be a part of Tarcher Perigee's community to bring positive change in this
world! See exclusive author videos, discover new and exciting books, learn
about upcoming events, connect with author blogs and websites, and more!
www.tarcherbooks.com

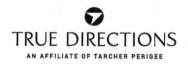

TRUE DIRECTIONS
AN AFFILIATE OF TARCHER PERIGEE